Other books  :

DAN   ͟LOVED
Resurrecting   ͟ᴛhrough Profound Relating

The sensual and sexual metaphor of Dancing with The Beloved may be challenging to accept as a metaphor for relating to the world and to your God. Yet this message of the sacred dance is a beautiful, poetic, and loving metaphor of relationship that can bring a personal revelation to those who are ready to receive it. It is the metaphor of profound relatedness found in the most traditional of Western mystical practices and one that can facilitate and catalyze a deeper, more sublime, and personal relationship with all those whom you love and, ultimately, with The Divine God. When The Divine is perceived as a lover or The Beloved instead of a stern, patriarchal Godhead, a new experience of intimacy and profound relatedness can be realized and unfolded in one's being, resulting in a deeper and more intimate relationship with the entire world—with all of life.

Dancing With The Beloved by Dr. Donovan has been described as "an excursion of profound thoughts on human existence."—*Ken Ostrander, Ed.D. Professor of Education, University of Washington*

THE FACE OF CONSCIOUSNESS
A Guide to Self-Identity and Healing

The Face of Consciousness offers a new perspective on consciousness and its manifestation as life. It proposes a theory that explains the "why" of creation and life and defines the transformational process of healing in a way in which it can be practically applied to one's life enabling one to transcend death and transform illness into greater life. This unifying theory is predicated upon the primary theme of self-realized identity. It is based on the properties of living systems, as described by modern physicists, biologists, philosophers and mystics. The fabric of this theory is woven from parallel threads of evidence based on the mystical traditions and scientific evidence pinpointing consciousness as the fundamental phenomenon (the "Materia Prima") of life and the conclusion that the primal driving force of life (its "raison d'etre") is its "sacred quest" for a sense of its own identity i.e., a realization of itself through the experience of itself. *The Face of Consciousness* was a finalist in the 2007 Nautilus Books Awards.

The Face of Consciousness has been called "A New Age Masterpiece" and described as "a bold and imaginative work, brilliantly researched, penetrating to the core of the question that confronts us all: Who are we? What are we?"—*Evan Harris Walker, Ph. D., Physicist and author of "The Physics of Consciousness" and founder of the Walker Cancer Institute*

FORTY YEARS
OF SACRED
SPACE

Life Lessons from a Doctor's Notebook

Dr. Patrick Donovan

BALBOA
PRESS

A DIVISION OF HAY HOUSE

To my many patients who have taught me so very much about life.

Balboa Press books may be ordered through booksellers or by contacting:

Balboa Press
A Division of Hay House
1663 Liberty Drive
Bloomington, IN 47403
www.balboapress.com
1 (877) 407-4847

Printed in the United States of America.

ISBN: 978-1-4525-8438-6 (sc)
ISBN: 978-1-4525-8440-9 (hc)
ISBN: 978-1-4525-8439-3 (e)

Library of Congress Control Number: 2013918425

Balboa Press rev. date: 10/29/2013

To my wife Taylor,
who has enlightened me to the skills of relationship
and has stood by me through my many leavings.
She is a light in my life.

To my first grandchild presently on the way,
my children Erin and Connor
and step son Alessandro,
may they live their life stories heroically.

Dedicated to Dr. William Mitchel
Thanks Bill for teaching us how to "be the medicine."

"Experience is not what happens to a man; it is what a man does with what happens to him."
—*Aldous Huxley, Texts & Pretexts: An Anthology With Commentaries*

Table of Contents

Preface

It has been said, experience is the greatest teacher of us all. I believe that to be true. I further believe when our experience is extensive enough and combined with the relevant education and trained observational skills of a professional, an invaluable wisdom and authority emerges in us as it has in me. After forty-three years of professional patient care spent with thousands of patients in the intimate and sacred space of compassionate listening, trained observation, and problem solving, I have gained an insight into the workings of the human psyche and the role it plays in the development of illness and emergence of healing. It is from this wisdom and insight that I have written this book.

It is my wisdom, insight, and experience from which I have drawn upon for this book and no one else's. It is therefore apt to be influenced by my own interpretations, perceptions, and colorations based upon my own personal experience of life and my patients' lives. If there are ideas with which you disagree, put them on a shelf in your heart and mind and let them set awhile . . . steep awhile. You may find it was my personal coloration or interpretation you didn't agree with at first, and not the underlying truth. Take what I say here and plug it into your own experiences, perceptions and interpretations; see what you come up with. Find your own truths from it. Think hard and ponder long upon what I share of my experience. My hope is that it can help you renew and/or reconstruct your own ideas of health, life, death, illness, and healing and their function and meaning in our lives. Although I am a Naturopathic Primary Care Physician and have forty-three years of professional patient care under my belt, I remain first and foremost an artist, poet, and philosopher. Therefore, this book is more a book of philosophical insights and poetic dialogue on health, healing and the nature of illness than it is a scientific tome. It isn't based on years of clinical research data and scientific studies. It isn't meant to be. It is meant to be human, organic, sensual, and real; an observational dialogue from the heart, mind and soul of an experienced and tempered care giver.

A poet, artist and philosopher at heart, I graduated from high school with a scholarship for art school. After two days at one of the best art colleges in the nation at the time, the Columbus College of Art and Design, I ended up telling the Dean of Students where to put my scholarship and it wasn't in a file drawer. We had a strong philosophical disagreement about the length of my hair and other sundry details about dress-codes and student housing. Needless to say, my sojourn in art school was quite brief and I walked out on my scholarship and my future as a professional artist.

After that experience, I then pursued my life-long passion of philosophy at Ohio State University. In the midst of my second quarter there, all hell broke loose on campus with major antiwar protests occurring on the same weekend as the famous Kent State University shootings occurred (Kent State students were shot and killed by National Guard soldiers on campus for protesting the war.). Things got horribly chaotic on the Ohio State University campus as well with bullets and tear gas canisters flying, buildings burning, students beaten, multiple streets blockaded for many blocks, and the campus closed down. I left in the middle of this craziness and walked out on my future dream as a professor of philosophy.

After a brief exploration of Ireland on foot with a guitar and back pack on my back, my life path took an unexpected ninety degree turn. I ended up graduating from college in 1976 with a registered nursing degree instead of a degree in art or philosophy. Life does these things to us you know . . . ninety degree turns when we least expect them because it has something different planned for us. Although I continued painting and writing poetry and music on my own time, I worked as a Registered Nurse and then later pursued a doctorate degree in Naturopathic Medicine and graduated from Bastyr University in Seattle, Washington in 1985.

I then devoted my life work to becoming the best physician and care giver I could turning my philosophical inquiring and artistic pursuits on to the human condition and its struggle with illness. While raising my two children (Erin and Connor) and establishing myself in the field of Naturopathic Medicine, I began to pursue my art, poetry and music again in a way that I could integrate them into my medicine and my patient care. As an artist, I always enjoyed working with the human form and the expression of the inner world of human emotion through both figure and portrait. This artistic exploration helped me in my clinical practice and healing work. It has given me a deeper understanding and insight into the formative and archetypal world of the human psyche and emotion. It also taught me that all healing is an act of creativity. As I state in my first book, *The Face of Consciousness,* "Creativity is 'the elixir of life' that heals and transforms life. Through the creative process you enter that sacred place, that 'zone of evolution' where the world lights up to itself as you light up to the world." Through the creative process we are healed.

My poetic musings and musical talents have also helped me in my patient care and practice of medicine as well as with the writing of this book. Through my poetry, I have gained a deeper comprehension of the importance of communication and dialogue in the establishment of the deep intimacy of "profound relatedness" and its relationship to healing. Much of my clinical work and writing involves intense and probing dialogue of a very intimate nature. As a musician and song writer, I have gained a greater appreciation for the rhythms of life and a deeper awareness of the sensual and harmonious nature of each soul's sacred dance of relationship. How well we do that dance is an essential aspect to our healing. So, dance well the transformative dance of profound relatedness and live authentically and creatively the Hero's journey as it takes you from illness into healing. But, more than anything, be the medicine you need and share it with the world.

Patrick Donovan,
September, 2013

Acknowledgements

This book is only possible because of the many patients whose lives I have had the honor to know, whose struggles I have had the privilege to witness and, whose stories have been entrusted to me to carry until the day I die. If I were to die tomorrow, I would pass from this life a rich man because of them. My wife Taylor is a brilliant internal consultant for a large health insurance firm. However, she is also my brilliant internal consultant and without our many "internal consults," this book would be so much less than it is. Thank you Taylor for the grammatical corrections as well. Then, there is my good friend Dan Cicora, his intelligent and insightful critiques of each chapter and our resultant MANY philosophical conversations have been invaluable to the quality of this book. Thank you Dan, for keeping my eye on the Fifteenth Century Italian philosophers. Thank you Lucy Vaughters, for your suggestions, support and initial edits. Our early conversations helped me realize I had something of value to share in this book. I must also acknowledge my office staff and partners (Lisa, Angie, Nancy, Dr. Mona, Dr. Steurich, and Dr. Fleetwood) for putting up with my many piles while I was working on this book. They have been invaluable at keeping me focused.

Finally, there are countless numbers of incredible physicians and health care providers with whom I have worked over the years who have taught me so well the skills of compassionately witnessing and care giving. Most importantly, I must acknowledge my mentor and friend, Dr. William Mitchel for teaching me how to BE the medicine. I so miss our many conversations about healing and life as we sat around the lunch table every week at Bastyr University. It always started off as the two of us but ended up with ten to twenty students gathered around us hungry for Bill's wisdom.

Chapter One

To Be Known

"Health is the functional result of a living system's
full engagement and participation in the process of
continuous creation for the purpose of self-revelation
and self-affirmation. It is not the absence of illness."
(*P. Donovan & H. Joinerbey: "The Face of Consciousness"*)

"The good physician treats the disease; the great
physician treats the patient who has the disease"
(*Sir William Osler*)

The Real Medicine

I have worked as a professional health care provider for more
than forty years immersed in the intimate, sacred space of
therapeutic relationship with my patients. Over this time, I
have learned a lot and have become acutely aware of an important
personal truth: Patients do not come to the doctor solely to be
cured; they come to be Known. The "real medicine" that heals
each one of us on the deepest of levels is not found in a pill, a food,
or an exercise alone. It is found in the discovery of ourselves. We
are healed in the realization of who we are and why we are here.

For us to taste this real medicine of self-discovery, we are
invited to risk our life for a fuller life. To experience its potency and
magic, we must be willing to slay dragons and apply penetrating
and purposeful introspection to our daily life so that we can
acknowledge and bless our successes and failures. To be healed

1

by this medicine is to experience our life as a revelation of itself because this medicine is one that is fashioned of self-revelation and self-transformation. Its actions are facilitated by our struggle to grow, evolve and self-affirm against the incessant drag of entropy and transform into a fuller realization of our self through the disintegrating trend of death and chaos we call illness.

Through my decades of patient care I have come to understand true healing to be a creative act of self-discovery and self-transformation made possible only by the transformative journey illness provides us. The 20th century philosopher and theologian, Paul Tillich tells us, "Healing is not healing, without the essential possibility and existential reality of illness."[1] I agree. Without illness, our healing could not happen. Illness makes our healing possible. It allows for the "essential possibility and existential reality" of our healing. I have witnessed that healing open my patients up to a greater emergence and awareness of themselves and the world around them. Further, our life is what provides us with the fertile soil for our healing to occur out of which our ultimate and full life story then emerges as its own revelation.

Illness as Healing

Any one of us taking the time to truly look at ourselves can readily see that our lives are a continuous experience of birth, death, and rebirth. I like to refer to this triumvirate of experiences as continuous creation. Through continuous creation, our life continually and creatively affirms and reaffirms itself repeatedly against the unremitting drag of ennui, stagnation, and sameness. It continuously reaffirms itself against the continuous demands of death looming always in the shadows of our life. As our life's architect, we are expected to endlessly create newness out of the archaic, novelty out of uniformity. We are always in a constant creative flux of change. As the Stoic philosopher, Marcus Aurelius has instructed, "Unceasingly contemplate the generation of all things through change, and accustom thyself to the thought that the nature of the universe delights above all in changing the things that exist and making new ones of the same pattern. For everything that exists, is the seed of that which shall come from it." Thus, we bear within ourselves the continual, eternal regeneration of the seed of our new life.

It is said, the only constant is change. The change required for our life's continuous creation and renewal of itself is self-transformation, hopefully a transformative change we have consciously acknowledged and chosen. Death is the transformational agent hidden within change. All life within the Creation requires of itself this transformational death for its rebirth, continuance and evolution just as all healing requires the disruptive dynamic of illness for its realization and fulfillment. When we think of it, death and illness are necessary catalysts in our lives; they provide us with the motivational constructs to transform, grow, adapt, and evolve. Through illness, death, and rebirth our life becomes a revelation of itself, a continuous yet fuller recreation of itself. As Pierre Teillard de Chardin would tell us, we continuously move toward the Omega Point. Healing, when we choose to pursue it, is always a transformational event and our life is a continuous series of these events. As we live, we are healed. The more fully we live our lives, the more completely we are healed. Healing, therefore, is an agent of our individual self-realization that transports us into a greater level of wholeness, integration, and completion.

Chaos and Change

Chaos, as described in the new theories of complexity and chaos, is the harbinger of change. It is the bringer of chance and opportunity. It heralds the beginning of the transformative process through death into new life and healing. As such; it is an inescapable reality of life yet, it is a necessary and welcome reality which beckons us toward growth, fulfillment, and ever expanding possibilities for healing. Chaos is found everywhere in nature as life struggles to survive and evolve against the disintegrating trend of entropy. To paraphrase N. Hall in *Exploring Chaos*, chaos stimulates the generation of new manifestations of complexity and diversity from tiny stimuli allowing us to evolve.[2] It deconstructs the existing order of our life, so the new, more complex, and more self-affirming order of a new "I" can emerge reconstructed from the ashes of the old "I." As Nobel Prize-winning physicist, Erwin Schrodinger describes, "At every step, on every day of our life, as it were, something of the shape that we possessed until then has to change, to be overcome, to be deleted and replaced by something new."[3] So, functioning as the transformative or chaotic element in our healing, illness is the root of our healing's creativity, the essence of our healing's beauty, and the purpose of our healing's liberation.

With this in mind, we might want to think much more carefully about the ramifications of *completely* removing or suppressing illness as it is addressed in our present healthcare system. The journey through our illness may be precisely the very experiential journey we need to realize our healing and to become something greater, to realize ourselves more fully. After all, we don't "get" cancer. We are not healthy one day and then get cancer the next day. Cancer, like any illness, is a process. We "become" our cancer over time as it becomes an expression of us.

We "are" the cancer we manifest. Our cancer arises out of our own tissue and cellular make up. To rid our self of our cancer is to rid our self of a part of our self. Instead of thinking about illness as something we "get," something separate from ourselves needing to be removed or defeated . . . as we do when we undertake the "war on cancer," we might well do better viewing our illness as a transformational journey that must be undertaken and completed for our healing to occur. This way we end up transforming our self into something more whole and complete instead of getting rid of a part of our self.

If we view our illness as such a journey, then the "true job" of a health care provider must be as an educated, intelligent and compassionate guide directing us through the chaos of our illness into the new order of wellness awaiting us at the completion of our healing journey. By understanding illness in this way, health care providers may quickly realize the important questions to be asked here of their patients. These questions are no longer solely focused upon, "How do I eliminate my patient's illness or help my patient fight it?" More significantly, the questions become, "What is it within my patient that needs to die . . . that needs to be sacrificed, released, and transformed?" and "What is it in my patient that needs to be reborn . . . what is it that needs to be facilitated and realized into a fuller manifestation?"

My personal observations over these many years of caring for people professionally has taught me that illness serves us by acting as life's destructive, disintegrating, and profaning process. I have come to appreciate illness as being absolutely crucial to our health as death is absolutely indispensable to life; just as the rotting wood and the decomposing debris on the forest floor is absolutely essential for the healthy growth and lushness of the forest's canopy. Health cannot exist without disease and our healing is impossible without the transformative opportunity the

5

chaotic struggle of illness offers us. Healing through our illness is our path toward greater Being.

We might further understand that all healing involves a risk, a sacrifice or loss of something, a death of some kind to transform and facilitate the rebirth of new life. Like the phoenix out of the ashes, something of the "old" order and function of who we have been, something of our life style, belief system and story must be let go and sacrificed in the transformative fire of illness in order to make way for our healing and "new" order of being. As Tilich informs us, "Life must risk itself to win itself, but in the risking it may lose itself. A life which does not risk disease . . . even in the highest forms of the life of the spirit, is a poor life, as is shown, for instance, by the hypochondriac or the conformist."[4] Our illness is the physical evidence of this sacrificial, transformative process occurring in our life. It is the evidence of our healing taking place. It becomes the very process through which we must pass to complete our healing journey. "Healing is not healing, without the essential possibility and existential reality of illness."[5] They are one and the same, just different sides of the same continuum.

The Dynamics of Illness

The extent to which we manifest our illness when caught in the state of our transformational chaos is directly related to:

1) Our initial *vitality* (the strength of our "vital force") and the potency of that vitality needed to propel us through the chaos of our illness;

2) The characteristics of the *triggering stimuli* (stressors; environmental exposures; dietary, genetic and life style risk factors; etc.) associated with the onset of our illness;

3) The *intensity of the chaos* causing our illness into which we have been plunged;

4) The *magnitude of resulting disorder* we undergo due to the illness; and

5) The *degree of rigidity and resistance* we have to the transformative change demanded of us through our illness process.

With these factors in mind, it becomes imperative for our healthcare providers to:

1) Assist us in maximizing our vital force;

2) Understand the characteristics of the risk factors and pathology underlying our illness;

3) Minimize or palliate the intensity of the chaos (pain and disability) that is underlying our illness and distracting us from our transformative work so as to facilitate our ability to more readily and consciously complete our healing journey;

4) Minimize the resulting disorder of our illness without suppressing the transformational process of it; and

5) Remove or reduce the obstacles obstructing our healing process on all levels.

This last factor is of particular importance to us on the psycho-emotional and spiritual levels. It is important to us here because it includes identifying, eliminating and resolving any of our self-destructive habits and lifestyles or restrictive beliefs and fears we have causing us to manifest rigidity and resistance to our healing. Oddly enough, I have found many of my patients through the years to be resistant to the transformative changes required for their healing. Some have even been in opposition to it. Further, so many of them even find it difficult or are fully unable to visualize their life as it could be if they were healed of their illness and no longer had to live under the restraints and limitations of their disease process. This aspect of human resistance has always been mind-boggling to me.

How can we not know or not be able to visualize and imagine what our life would be like without our illness? What would prohibit this? Why would any of us, in the depths of our struggle and suffering with illness, not want to at least try to visualize ourselves in a better place surrounded by loving friends, family and natural beauty doing the creative things we most enjoy doing? As I have witnessed far too often, fear is the common culprit here. I have observed so much of our lives to be directed by our fears: the fear of loosing anything even for the possibility of gaining something new and different ("fear of risking death for new life"); the fear of realizing our own power and our own light; the fear of assuming responsibility for ourselves and/or others; the fear of accountability for our own feelings, thoughts, actions, and words and; the fear of dying as well as the fear of living.

I think for many of us, we are more fearful of change than we would like to believe. We fear letting go of what is familiar and routine, of letting go of the experience to which we have come to self-identify as "our reality" even if it is based on illusion. We fear letting go of it more than holding on to it even if it has become an obstacle to our healing and fuller self-realization. As the saying goes, "We would rather wrestle with the devil we know." This is where the rigidity and resistance to change plays its part in keeping us ill. We would rather hold on to the burning, sinking boat than risk letting go of it to swim to shore even if the shore is a short distance away. Our human psyche is programmed by our ego mind to believe what is familiar to us is safe and what is unknown to us is dangerous. This is where our life must risk itself to find itself.

Here is where our asking the appropriate questions can reveal what must be risked and lost and what must be found and realized into manifestation so our healing may occur. I have witnessed the answers to these questions hiding in the nature of our illness; in the nature of our symptoms, signs, and underlying pathology. It is here where the story of our transformative change is continually being told and the answers to our healing are persistently revealed. It is important for our health care providers and for all of us to be able to read our story through our signs and symptoms. By understanding the story of our illness, we can better realize the course and direction of our healing and the guidance needed to be given to us so as to help us fulfill our journey into healing.

The Story of Illness Is the Story of Healing

I have taken the complete medical, psycho-social, and familial "histories" of thousands of patients through these many years of my naturopathic medical practice. In listening to these histories, I have discovered an interesting truth: *the story of our life reveals the story of our illness and the story of our illness reveals the story of our life.* The theme of our life's struggles and the resistance we manifest to the transformational changes demanded of us by those struggles is the theme that commonly plays itself out in our illness's pathology and symptoms. The morphogenetic field of our consciousness (our conscious and unconscious thoughts, feelings, dreams, and desires as well as our familial genetics) is the form matrix that dictates and directs the underlying cellular and biochemical patterning of who we are as we manifest physically in this third dimensional existence. If our morphogenetic consciousness matrix is dysfunctional in any way, so will be its physical outcomes on our cellular make up and physical functions. In this way, the field

9

of our consciousness can dictate the physical form and cellular expression of our illness.

So many of the stories of illness I have heard begin with a single psycho-emotional "wounding" event or with multiple wounding experiences over time that carry within them the same general theme of trauma and dysfunction. We all appear to have our own individual experience(s) of wounding. However, many if not most of our woundings involve primary archetypal themes shared by all of us in our "collective unconscious," as famously described by the psychologist, Carl Jung. We experience wounding as some form of a violation to our intrinsic and authentic sense of who we are as a conscious individual and to our intrinsic expectation and understanding of what it means to love and to be loved and valued as an individual. We feel and experience this wound deep in the consciousness matrix of our being as it breaks the fundamental relationships that form the fabric of our human existence. As a result, "our intrinsic, authentic sense of self is plunged into the experience of annihilation and nonbeing."[6]

According to John Firman and Ann Gila, from their book *The Primal Wound*, "However this wound is inflicted, it is a break in the intricate web of relationships in which we live, move, and have our being. A fundamental trust and connection to the universe is betrayed, and we become strangers to ourselves and others, struggling for survival in a seemingly alien world."[7] I have watched that struggle for survival emerge from the source of our wounding to become the story that dictates the identity construct and interpersonal dynamics of who we are and who we become. It becomes the theme pattern imprinted upon the deep unconsciousness matrix of our cellular and psycho-social identity that directs the unfolding of our life. As I have said repeatedly, "Our issues are in our tissues". From here, the theme pattern of our wounding directs the telling of our story and choreographs our life dance. We dance our wounds just as we dance our celebrations. They never leave us no matter how many years of therapy we may undergo. They just become part of our dance choreographed into the rhythms of our life. We are our woundings just as we are our celebrations, only we can decide how we choose to live them.

The story of our "struggle for survival in a seemingly alien world," unconsciously formulated from our wounding experience, is a false story or a half-truth at best in the greater scheme of what our soul intrinsically knows is "a loving Universe" where we are all connected. It is a partially fictional story made up from an unintentional error in our emotional interpretation of an event or events. So many of our wounding stories sound like this: "I am not good enough." "I am not loved." "I am all alone." "I always screw up and can't do anything right." "I am a 'bad' person." This is because, as Firman and Gila write, ". . . a fundamental trust and connection to [a loving] Universe has been betrayed, and we become strangers to ourselves and others." These partially fictional stories of estrangement and betrayal are eventually played out in our life and lived as self-fulfilling prophecies. When read correctly, these stories can be witnessed in the symptoms and pathological characteristics of our illness and can, therefore, offer deep insight into the causative energetics of our illness and the healing direction needed for us to take.

For instance, when our underlying energetic story is one of anger and blame as a result of our deeper feelings of alienation and betrayal, the pathology of this energetic story is commonly displayed as inflammation. If that anger is directed at "self," ("I hate myself." or "I hate what I do.") and we become highly self-critical and self-deprecating, we may well exhibit the inflammatory pattern of autoimmunity ("self, attacking self" or "me, attacking myself") where our immune system is turned against our "self" proteins and attacks our own tissues. Further, if our anger and negative self-criticism is focused on the results of our actions, work performance, or athletic performance for instance, we may present with an autoimmune arthritic or neurological condition such as rheumatoid arthritis (R.A.) or multiple sclerosis (M.S.). These disorders then conveniently limit us and prohibit us from successfully performing the very work/actions in question. The outcome of our resulting illness then serves us in a negative way. It ends up protecting us from "screwing up" and having to endure our further self-criticism and self-directed anger because of our perceived "screw up." Ironically, however, it then also becomes a self-fulfilling prophecy, i.e. "I can't do anything right because I have R.A. or M.S." Our illness becomes our convenient excuse. In this illness scenario, the appropriate questions to ask are: "How does our illness negatively serve ourselves?" and "How does our illness display the underlying story of our wounding?" What is the healing journey to self-transformation and self-actualization hidden in our illness story?

Identity and Meaning

When we ask ourselves the insightful and appropriate questions regarding the dynamics of our illness, our healing journey begins. It is a journey that eventually becomes the story of our life as well as the story of our healing. It becomes our "hero's journey" with us as the hero or heroine on an exploratory quest into the depths of our wounding, into the depths of our subconscious to discover the answers to the questions begged by the dynamics of our illness. For us to find the answers to these probing questions, a wholehearted and profound introspection and a willingness to risk death for new life is demanded of us. The answers, like the

Holy Grail, when found, will revitalize us and reawaken us to the obstacles obstructing our healing process. They will reveal to us our individual path to greater self-realization, self-actualization and healing.

The obstacles to our healing include our self-destructive habits and lifestyles as well as the restrictive beliefs and fears causing our rigidity and resistance to transformative change. With perseverance and self-sacrifice, we can overcome these obstacles and transform them into life-sustaining practices and processes that promote our healing, wholeness and personal transformation. With another "particular medicine" as well, available from our health care practitioner, this transformation is made even more possible. This medicine can only be administered via the therapeutic relationship of a trained healthcare provider. However, it is only curative when the provider is compassionate, nonjudgmental and professionally engaged and fully present with us in the sacred space of profound relating. Being present in this way, in that sacred space, our story can be safely revealed and through it, we can be truly "seen," truly witnessed, and truly known.

In my witnessing of so many life stories, I have come to understand that Life, as it manifests in all of its many diverse forms and expressions has, at its very core of existence, an agenda, a "prime directive" for us if you will. That prime directive is for it (Life) to be all it can be to its fullest and most diverse manifestations of itself. Since we are one of life's many expressions, its prime directive also applies to us and is also at the very core of our own existence. It drives our self-affirming need to BE and to be all that we were born to be to our fullest and further, to be seen and witnessed in our BE-ingness. We are here to live our story and have it known to our self and to others.

The story of our journey through illness to a new self-realization of healing is further catalyzed by asking the essential questions of identity and meaning: "Who am I?" and "Why am I here?" Our answering of these questions activates the "real medicine" found here in this query. Our questions of identity and meaning are familiar questions to us all. Most of us know them very well. They regularly, consciously cry out from the midst of our preadolescent and adolescent woundings and haunt the intimacy of every meaningful interaction and relationship we have. More often we ignore them or actively suppress them within the shadows of our subconscious because answering them is a frightening proposition! It means we will have to acknowledge and live our full potential powerfully and authentically. Most of us choose instead to battle with the feelings of anxiety, depression, failure, fear, loneliness, and isolation that arise from their suppression and denial . . . feelings I have commonly witnessed as causatively associated with illness and overwhelmingly present in the lives of the majority of my patients.

I believe we all come into the experience of life to be known to ourselves and to others. Through this act of knowing ourselves and being known, we are given meaning and made whole again. Through this act of knowing ourselves and being known we are healed. This may be why the ancient directive on the Temple of Apollo at Delphi reads, "Know Thyself." Asking the essential questions of self-identity and meaning demands of us the willingness and fortitude to "know ourselves" and to manifest and experience the answers fully in our lives. Discovering who we are is not a singular, momentary revelational event. It is the activity of our life and the reason why we are here. It takes continual, profound, intense introspection and examination of our lives. As Socrates wrote, "The unexamined life is not worth living." I say a life of personal and social illiteracy and anonymity is not worth living.

References

1. Tilich P. *The Meaning of Health*. North Atlantic Books, Berkley, 1981
2. Hall N (Ed.): *Exploring Chaos*. Norton & Company, N.Y.,1991
3. Schrodinger E: *What Is Life?* N.Y., Cambridge University Press, 1992; 100
4. Tilich P. *The Meaning of Health*. 1981
5. Ibid.
6. Firman J & Gila A: *The Primal Wound: A Transpersonal View of Trauma, Addiction and Growth*. State University of New York Press, 1997; 2
7. Ibid.

Chapter Two

Living the Prime Directive

"Each incarnation has a potentiality, and the
mission of the life is to live that potentiality."
(*Joseph Campbell, The Power of Myth, 1988*)

"Do not follow where the path may lead. Go instead
where there is no path and leave a trail."
(*Ralph Waldo Emerson, The Selected
Writings of Ralph Waldo Emerson*)

The Prime Directive

In the spring of 2003, I was sitting in a circle of professors and students from Bastyr University. As an adjunct professor at the University at that time, I was then engaged in a workshop with faculty and students at the Whidbey Island Institute. It was a three-day workshop involving personal transformation for the students lead by several faculty members. At the end of the third day, while we were all in a circle for the closing ceremony, this question was posed to each of us: "What is your primary responsibility to yourself and to your community of life?" Based upon each person's answer to that question, we were each to make a promise to ourselves and to the community present as to how we would fulfill our personal responsibility.

Of course I was intrigued with the question both for myself and for the young students in the circle. As I watched their faces deeply pondering their answers, I found myself also lost in deep thought about the answer. I was not just reviewing the weekend's many intimate conversations and dialogues as I expected, but contemplating my life on so many levels. Just what is my primary responsibility to myself, to my family, friends and community . . . to life itself? Lost in this contemplative inner exploration, I suddenly found myself catapulted back into the present . . . actually shaken to my very roots from an answer given by one of my colleagues, Dr. Rowen Hamilton. Upon his turn to answer, Dr. Hamilton stood up in a very purposeful yet humble manner and gently, but profoundly said, "Above all, I have a responsibility to be who I was born to be in my fullest." After a momentary pause, he then promised to be "that person" and quietly sat down.

A soberingly powerful and intensely present silence overcame the circle. The proverbial "pin" could have been heard; in the midst of this silence was a pregnant space spanning what seemed many minutes. It was as though the voice of destiny had just spoken directly to our souls. The simplicity and pure honesty of his answer left each one of us awe-struck and speechless as we considered the intrinsic directive: "*To be who we are born to be in our fullest!*" It seemed as if this directive had shattered all delusional constructs and preconceived notions any of us had about ourselves and what our lives were about. I could see the impact his answer had on the faces of everyone in that circle. It had stopped each one of us dead in our tracks, but why? Why was this simple, honest reply to the question posed so profoundly affecting us? Was there something deep in our inner nature, in our soul memory that resonated with and understood the fundamental truth of Dr. Hamilton's answer? It certainly embraced some of the greatest concerns of human existence and deeper mysteries of being that have continued for centuries to confound us all, even the greatest of philosophers and theologians; mysteries such as consciousness and self-awareness, destiny and fate, free-will and predetermination.

The renowned story teller and mythologist Michael Meade, in his book *Fate And Destiny*, tells the traditional story of Rabbi Zushya. Rabbi Zushya was a wise and famous Jewish mystic and teacher who, on his death bed, was afraid to meet God because he was concerned he could not answer God's only question: "Zushya, why were you not more like Zushya?" In other words, God was asking Zushya if Zushya was what he was born to be in his fullest. Why did this concern Zushya so? He was wise and supposedly knew all the great mysteries of God and life. How did he not know the answer to God's question? Can any one of us ever know the answer? As Meade writes, "Every life must eventually become a revelation of itself."[1] Is your life "becoming a revelation of itself?" How would you answer God if you died today and God asked you, "While you lived your life, did you become what you were born to be in your fullest?" Do you know yourself well enough and do you have some sense or vision of your own destiny well enough to identify an answer?

As I further considered Dr. Hamilton's response, I began to realize the primal truth of its directive. In reality, all any one of us can ever be is the person we are and the life we live as that person "eventually becomes the revelation of itself." In other words, I realized there is no "right" or "wrong" way of being myself. I AM the revelation of myself! By virtue of my own separate, individual uniqueness formed and shaped by my genetic code, familial patterns, and personal life experiences, any expression of myself is the "right" expression because it is simply me being who I AM. Therefore, the only promise I can ever responsibly make with some sense of honest conviction is to be who I AM, or is it? This begged my further inquiry. Is the "who I AM" enough or is there a deeper meaning implied? Is there an imminent sense of destiny insinuated in the person I was born to be as opposed to just being who I AM? The essential question in my mind came to be: Is there something more I am to become other than just who I AM . . . something destined? As I explored this question, I quickly realized I did know one thing. "Who I AM" is clearly a dynamic ever evolving identity influenced by a multitude of factors at any one moment.

Self-identity, for any self-aware being, is constantly evolving and adapting from one moment to the next. It is in a continuous state of being formed, shaping and reshaping itself while being hourly sculpted by fate's creative hand via a combination of numerous external forces and influences (social, familial, political, environmental etc.) combined with our internal reactions to those external forces and influences. Yet, I felt as though there was still something more deep inside of me, something constant and unchanging at the very core of "who" I AM . . . something of "my" nature, of "my" self-identity that made me unique and different than anyone else in spite of so many shared human commonalities and experiences. Further, I felt as though "the something constant at my core" is always calling out to me, beckoning me in some strange and haunting way, like a light house in the fog of night directing me through the perilous seas of my fate to some yet unseen but strangely familiar port of destiny only I could recognize. This is true for us all. In spite of our shared commonalities, something makes us distinctively different in our own inimitable way. If we listen carefully, we can hear that uniqueness as it calls out to us to follow its beckoning light to the harbor of our own particular destiny . . . to the secret place of our own particular gifts and individuality. I believe it is this uniqueness and individuality of life's many forms, life's myriad of diversity that makes life so interesting, rich and beautiful with its interplay of individually unique characters, qualities and species and its many exotic harbors.

At the time this workshop was taking place, it just so happened I was in the midst of writing my first book, *The Face of Consciousness*. I had just finished writing a section on diversity and self-identity. So, the idea of each one of us being unique and responsible to be who we were born to be intrigued me. It was fully in sync with all I had been studying and writing about regarding the nature of consciousness, self-identity and living systems. Every living system is a unique, individual whole unto itself and is made up of parts that are also unique, individual wholes made up of other parts, and so on. According to science writer and philosopher, Arthur Koestler, every whole is a part and every part is a whole, each unique. Since every part is also a whole unto itself and visa versa, Koestler referred to everything as a "holon." He described every living system as a "holon" possessed of two opposite tendencies: a tendency to integrate as part of a larger whole, and a self-assertive tendency to preserve its individual autonomy and uniqueness as a whole unto itself.[2] Could that "self-assertive tendency" be the "something constant at the core" in each one of us that calls out to us and guides us through our life's story, through the perils of our fated seas to the unique harbor of our own distinctive destiny guarantying life its diversity?

As the biological sciences have clearly witnessed, the more diverse a living system is (the more unique and autonomous are its parts), the more robust and healthy is that system. Diversity is a special form of creativity and appears to be a primary directive of life because it assures the maximal unfolding of all the possibilities of identity and relationship life has to offer.[3] Life's preponderance for diversity assures the maximal unfolding of the distinct and peculiar characteristics of the full potential of each one of us as individual holons. As I think about it, the U.S.

Army (Who would have thought?) actually had it right: "Be all that you can be." Above all, life wants each one of us "to be all that we can be."

Know Thyself

If I AM who I AM and I AM a unique individual as is each one of us, what is the "constant at my core" that makes me unique? Is it my genes? Some might say it is. But, according to the human genome project, genetically we are more alike than different, even between different geographical and racial populations. According to research appearing in the science journal Genetics, "The proportion of human genetic variation due to differences between populations is modest, and individuals from different populations can be genetically more similar than individuals from the same population."[4] Research in genetics has also shown we share 98% of our human DNA with chimpanzees. 98% of our DNA is identical to a chimpanzee's DNA![5] Not so hard for me to believe when I think of a few friends I had as a teenager. As a matter of fact, researchers finished mapping the genome of the domestic dog and the results showed, among other things, that dogs, mice, and humans share a core set of DNA. Obviously, it isn't genetics alone that contributes to uniqueness. What makes me different from you, different from anyone else, even from a chimpanzee or a dog, for that matter, is something more . . . something of cumulative life-experience and of the deep self. It exists at a more profound and fundamental level than biology and genetics alone. It is something of consciousness and self-awareness . . . something of the soul.

When Moses encountered God as the burning bush on Mount Sinai and received the Ten Commandments, according to the biblical account in King James version, Exodus 3:13-14, Moses asked God, "When I come unto the children of Israel, and shall say unto them, The God of your fathers hath sent me unto you; and they shall say to me, 'What is his name?' What shall I say unto them?" God replied, "I AM that I AM." I believe this name of God given to Moses by God represents the most basic, self-reflective statement of being possible. The word "*that*" appearing within God's name, is a linguistic symbol for the universal phenomenon of self-reflection that allows the self to behold itself. It acts as the mirror reflecting the image of I AM back to I AM allowing God to experience God so that God may know God. It allows God to, as Psalm 8:1 declares, "Behold the magnificence and glory of the Lord" and proclaim "How excellent is thy name in all the earth who has set thy glory above the heavens." As I have described with great detail in *The Face of Consciousness,* the creative, self-reflective act represented by God's name is intrinsic to all living systems and is essential for the development of self-awareness and self-consciousness. It not only allows the unrealized potential of life to fully manifest, affirm and eventually witness and realize all aspects of its beingness, but it also allows each one of us to do the same. It allows ourselves to experience ourselves that we may know ourselves.

For any of us to be "who we were born to be in our fullest" we must first know who we are at our core on a deep *soulular* level. Of course, this takes thorough, intense introspection and examination of one's life. As Socrates advised, "The unexamined life is not worth living." Of course it isn't! Without daily examination of one's life, it is difficult to evaluate the strange twists of fate we encounter and the outcomes of our choices and directions taken in response to those "strange twists." As Michael Meade tells us in his book, *Fate And Destiny*:

"Fate and the soul are woven of the same threads and fate includes the strange twists that make each soul unique and each life unpredictable. Denying all sense of fate and limitations in life also means denying any sense of inherent uniqueness in the soul. Our 'uniqueness' is woven exactly where the thread of destiny entwines with the twists of fate."[6]

The thread of destiny is that light beacon that guides us through the perilous seas of our fated life to our own unique harbor of *who* we are to be. It "entwines the twists of fate" at the points where we are confronted by potential navigational hazards forcing us to make directional changes (choices) based on avoidance or confrontation of those potential hazards. Therefore, the story of who we are first begins to be discovered within the story of our choices. The history of those choices throughout our life is the map of our life . . . the fingerprint of our identity. Without such information, the perilous sea of life is difficult to navigate. To know one's self is not an easy task. It is an ongoing process . . . a continual discovery and unfolding until one's life "becomes its own revelation of itself," as Meade writes. To know one's self is to know one's direction . . . to recognize and follow that directional beacon of light that helps us navigate the perils of fate's entwinements with destiny so that we may arrive at the harbor of our life's revelation of itself. To know one's self means also to understand our choices, how they empower us to become that which we are born to be, or how they may inhibit our growth and development and impede our possibility to move into the fullest expression of our potential. As the ancient inscription on the Temple of Apollo at Delphi reads, "Know Thyself." This, I firmly believe, is the most important of all life's directives.

Without knowing ourselves, it is difficult to be the person we were born to be.

As I sat in the circle with my students and colleagues that day considering further Dr. Hamilton's declaration and resultant promise, I realized I do have a responsibility to Life itself, as does every person living on this planet or in this universe. Our shared, primary responsibility to Life is to be the "unique, autonomous holon" we were born to be in our fullest and to do so means each one of us must know who we are at our core and be true to that self by fully realizing its potential. Like Polonius's last bit of advice to his son Laertes, in Shakespeare's Hamlet, "This above all, to thine own self be true." By so doing, we assure Life its maximal unfolding . . . its richness, robustness and diversity. By so doing, we can live our full potential and assure ourselves our destiny. But, there was yet one more responsibility I began to see emerging from all of this analytical ruminating. We have another responsibility to each other . . . to each living thing. It is the responsibility to allow each one of us to be that unique, autonomous holon we are each meant to be by ensuring and encouraging the freedom of expression for each one of us to do so. Each one of us has a story to tell . . . a life to live so that it can become its own revelation of itself.

By the time it was my turn to answer that day, I had realized there was another promise I had to make besides the promise to be *who* I was born to be in my fullest. It was the only promise I thought could respectfully follow such a primary promise as Dr. Hamilton's. I promised to encourage, support and inspire each one of the people present in that circle that day to become who they were born to be in their fullest and to refrain from obstruction or interference with their freedom to do so. Voltaire in his sagacity wrote: "I may not agree with what you have to say, but I'll defend to the death your right to say it." I understand that as a primary responsibility to be who I was born to be in my fullest, I also have a secondary responsibility to assure everyone else their individual freedom to be who they were born to be in their fullest, as well, even if I may not agree with the "who" they choose to be. Each of us has our own individual path and hidden gifts to discover and bring into the world. Each one of us is a unique individual expression of life's diverse nature of God being God and we have that story to tell.

At the moment I made my promise, one more thought occurred to me. It occurred to me what the "founding fathers" of the United States may have been trying to accomplish in the framing of the American Constitution. I believe they were constitutionally delineating the two fundamental responsibilities we have to ourselves and to each other: 1) to be what each one of us was born to be in our fullest; 2) to allow and assure all others the freedom to be what they were born to be in their fullest. The writers of the constitution were also attempting to construct the guidelines to preserve the freedoms and individual rights it would take to allow those responsibilities to be realized by each individual and the communities within which they lived. What a revelation it was to me to finally understand the depth of thought and insight it took for these founding fathers to construct the framework of democracy and individual freedoms upon which this country was built. I have come to realize these two fundamental responsibilities we have to ourselves and to each other are fundamental responsibilities shared by all conscious, self-aware beings throughout the universe.

Self-Aware and Self-Conscious

To "know yourself" and "be who you were born to be," requires self-awareness and the consciousness from which such self-awareness arises. If we think of it, self-awareness is fundamentally an awareness of our "self" as separate. Ironically, however, having an awareness of our self as separate automatically predicates awareness within us of something more . . . the awareness of something other than or outside of our self. That something we are aware of is "the other." An awareness of "the other" automatically infers an awareness of those attributes making us distinctly different from the other. As I explained in, *The Face of Consciousness,* The development of self-consciousness and identity is wholly dependent on an act of severance giving way to maximal contrast and the conscious illusion of separateness. We could say self-awareness is pretty much dependent upon the conscious realization of separateness and the ability to discriminate and differentiate between . . . to compare and contrast self and the other.

How do we know our selves or know we are separate individuals if we don't differentiate ourselves from others by comparing and contrasting ourselves with them? We might certainly consider checking ourselves out in a mirror if there is any question or confusion on our part as to who we are. Is that our face? Is that our body? (Maybe not, it might be looking a little too fat today to be ours!) If we confirm it's our face and our body, the next important question might be this: "Is that me in there behind those eyes and inside that body?" We could reply as Descartes might have replied to such a question if he were still alive: "I think I am in there, therefore I AM!" Or, we may have no way of knowing for sure until we make a few faces and perform a few gestures. "Yep, that's me. It's my face, my body, and it all works as I will it to work."

But is that really YOU? Is the "YOU" just that face and a body or is it more? If we are more than just a face, then what makes us more? What truly defines us . . . makes us different from anyone else? Who is that person inside the mirror and inside of each one of us making the faces and the gestures? Are we a single me or are we made up of many "me holons" . . . the moody holon; the pragmatic, impulsive, angry, and passive holons, and so forth, integrated into a whole person? Are we each a community made up of many cellular holons? One thing for sure is this, we are who we see in the mirror because our genes dictated or transcribed us to be so. But, since we share 98% of our genes with Chimpanzees and even more with our human neighbors, friends and family, it can't be the genes alone that make us who we are and give us our distinctive, individual characteristics.

If it isn't our genetics alone that makes us who we are, then what else is there that truly defines us as who we were born to be? Ultimately, I think it is our life story that describes and defines us best. That story *is* the story of our journey on the path of our own destiny as we have chosen and continue to choose to live it; *choice* being the primary factor.

References

1. Meade M: *Fate And Destiny: The Two Agreements of the Soul.* Greenfire Press, 2010, 82
2. From Arthur Koestler's book, *Janus: A Summing Up* as it appears excerpted in Barlow C (Ed.) *From Gaia to Selfish Genes. Cambridge*, MA: MIT Press, 1998, 91
3. According to physicist Fritjof Capra, the ability to generate configurations that are unique and constantly new is creativity and this creativity is a key property of all living systems. A

special form of this creativity is diversity. (Donovan P & Joiner Bey H: *The Face of Consciousness: A Guide to Self-Identity and Healing.* Lucky Press, 2006, 152-154)

4. Witherspoon DJ, et al: "Genetic Similarities Within and Between Human Populations." *Genetics.* 2007 May; 176(1): 351-359
5. Lovgren S: "Dog Genome Mapped, Shows Similarities to Humans." *National Geographic News.* Dec 7, 2005
6. Meade M: *Fate And Destiny: The Two Agreements of the Soul.* 2010, 2

Chapter Three

The One Thing

"Each one of us is concurrently a singular answer to life's
query of itself ("Who am I?") connected to all the other
possible answers. Every moment we live, every choice we make
formulates the reply. We are life's story being told every day.
(*P. Donovan & H. Joinerbey: The Face of Consciousness, 2006*)

"To live in hearts we leave behind is not to die."
(*Thomas Campbell*)

The Wonderful Blessing

I have been a professional healthcare provider for a little over
forty years now. I have been an Emergency Medical Technician
(E.M.T), a Registered Nurse (R.N.) and a Naturopathic
Doctor (N.D.). During that time, I have worked in an inner city
emergency room; in an infectious diseases intensive care and
post op open-heart surgical unit; in general, open-heart, vascular,
orthopedic, and plastic surgery; on numerous medical-surgical
floors at various major hospitals and; in multiple outpatient care
settings. The last twenty eight of those forty years I have spent in
private practice as a Naturopathic Primary Care Physician while
periodically serving as an adjunct Clinical Professor of Medicine
at Bastyr University. Throughout this time, I have seen more
than I would have liked, wept more than I could have imagined,
been responsible for more human lives than I could shoulder, held
more hands of strangers than I would have ever thought possible,

and heard the intricate details of more life stories than an average person hears in two lifetimes. More poignantly, I have watched the lives of too many heroic people slowly fade away and end in front of me after coming to know them and their life stories and feeling helpless in my ability to save them.

Of course, this experience is not something unique to me alone. It is what health care providers experience and do all the time. We providers share in this wonderful blessing of nearly daily participation in the more profound aspects of the human experience and its vast narrative of unique stories. Being allowed access into the deepest and most intense and sacred places of another person's life at a time of that person's greatest loss, vulnerability and pain is a most blessed gift. Anyone who is invited can go. It is an invitation into the more sublime and mysterious places of the human soul where the dragons of chaos reside and the shadows of death eternally dance their Shiva-like dance of destruction and resurrection. Of course, any one of us who is invited can enter these deep places of the human soul. We just need to put down our "smartphones," turn off our televisions, unplug our headsets, and close our laptops and *be* present in that deep place with a friend or loved one who needs to be witnessed in his/her struggle.

In these deep and sacred places, spirit is alive and magic happens. Life is most "real" here, more malleable and receptive to the transformative hands of change. So, it is in these sacrosanct places of so much struggle and loss where our lives are transformed through the death that reaffirms life. It is here also where our healing begins because, "All healing requires a death of some kind."[1] For healing to occur, something of the old must die so that something new can be born . . . can emerge out of the ashes of an old way of being.

It is a privilege for anyone to be invited by another into these secret places of the heart and soul to witness and participate in the more painful and hidden struggles of another person's life journey. It is a privilege that should never be taken lightly. It has taught me much and, at times, has shaken me to the very roots of my existence as it forced me to look at my own nakedness, dance with my own shadows, and slay my own dragons. Being invited into these secret places is like entering the inner sanctum of some great temple, like entering the "Holy of Holies" where the mystery of life presides and "The Face" of the divine is revealed in the face of another. In this place of profound relating, God lives and Spirit dances in the light of its own self-reflective revelation of itself. In this place also resides the Holy Grail of our own existence, the cup of our own unique blood essence forever intermixing and running over with the waters of life. Anyone can enter here with the appropriate invitation from another, but in here, honor, respect and humility are required while judgment is left at the door. People are naked here, vulnerable here, their most honest here. It is best for us to be prudent and discreet in this place for as we enter within and witness another's spirit dancing in the light of its own revelation, so do we witness that person's shadow.

Shadow Dancing

We do not see our shadows easily by the very definition and understanding of the "shadow aspect" of personality as described in Jungian psychology. Our shadow is the cumulative aspects of our deeper unconscious of which our conscious ego is not, and most often, chooses not to be fully conscious or aware. Our conscious ego mind perceives the shadow aspect of our consciousness as something less than desirable . . . in some cases even ugly, frightening, and despicable. Because our shadow is irrational and linked to the more primitive "animal instincts" of our survival and procreation, and because it arises out of the pain of our woundings, our ego believes our shadow and its elements of wounding are something to be hidden. So, they get stuffed away in the deep recesses of our unconscious mind where we can deny their existence and not have to deal with them. But, this stuffing activity eventually leads to a pressure-cooker effect of feelings, memories and emotions that, when released, express themselves as our illness story.

The more we pack our shadow elements away in our deep unconscious, the more energy it takes to keep them there. They are like little children or caged animals, always demanding of us our attention or pacing their cages anxious to be set free. The irony here is they are dynamic aspects of our own selves . . . of our lives, aspects desperately vital to the wholeness of who we are. As such, they are always anxious to be seen, heard, felt, and experienced. Keeping our shadow elements repressed, hidden and caged away in the depths of our unconscious mind fractionates the whole of who we are and gets to be very draining upon our physical and psycho-emotional well-being and conscious focus over time. The energetic demands put upon us by this repression become immense. Hence, the more we stuff our shadow elements down, the more we become exhausted and cognitively drained. Also, the more we suppress them, the more they push back, the more the pressure builds up for their need to be expressed and fully integrated into our conscious awareness. That pressure must be relieved healthfully. Little children must be held and loved and caged animals must be fed, watered and eventually set free. As I have seen in so many of my years of practice, if our shadow elements keep getting, repressed, ignored and not healthfully worked through and integrated into the "fullness" of our being by our conscious processing, they end up blowing holes in our conscious defenses from the pressure of their suppression and then either slowly leak out or gush out as illness affecting both our mind and body.

One way our shadow elements commonly leak out of their hiding places and begin to make themselves known to our conscious mind is through the psychological defense mechanism known as "projection." Projection is a defense mechanism we use to unconsciously reject our shadow elements, our own unacceptable attributes and resultant emotional responses from our woundings. We do this by ascribing them to objects or persons other than ourselves in the outside world instead of acknowledging them in their original source, in ourselves. In other words, we project the qualities of and the blame for our own shadow elements and woundings onto someone or something else. We then stand in criticism and judgment of that person or thing for having those shadow qualities and/or we persecute them for hurting us in the style and manner of our original wounding even though they had nothing to do with it. Most often, projection is the only way the majority of us can ever begin to experience our own unacceptable attributes and realize the theme of our wounding without having to feel the cutting pain of our own self-judgment, accountability, and ego-embarrassment. My father used to say, "Tell me what irritates you most about another and I will tell you all about yourself." So, we must be humble and prepared when we intimately witness another's dance and confront their shadow. It may not be "their" shadow we end up confronting.

Unfortunately, as long as we are caught in this self-defensive act of projective denial it becomes difficult to be accountable to and responsible for our own shadow elements, our own unacceptable attributes, feelings, and actions when we encounter them in ourselves. Without accountability and responsibility for our own actions and feelings, we become victims. Without recognizing the source of our wounding and the shadow themes unfolding behind the scenes of our story, it becomes much more difficult for us to healthfully engage and successfully transform them from the story of our illness into the story of our healing, the story of our self-transformation and self-realization. Without accountability and responsibility for and to ourselves, we are left feeling powerless, without personal integrity, at the mercy of the outside world proclaiming repeatedly: "It isn't my fault. It is someone else's fault!" "It is their fault!" "It is his or her fault!" "I can't do anything about it because I was hurt in this or that particular way."

With this scenario at work in our consciousness, apathy and ennui set in like dry rot. Our life story then becomes partially lived instead of fully lived. It also then becomes a story of victimization and powerlessness and not one of revelation and self-affirmation. Once this becomes the reality matrix of our life story, anything of truth or love that comes along seeming to fracture our matrix is rejected quickly by our self-protective ego mind. We see only what we want to see; hear only what we want to hear; believe only what we want to believe even when the "facts" dispute our belief. As Paul Simon wrote in his song, *The Boxer*, "All lies in jest, still a man hears what he wants to hear and disregards the rest." In my experience, I have found most of us find it difficult to even see the truth or recognize love when it knocks at our door or is offered to us. This is because it IS outside the realm of our reality matrix. This failure to recognize the apparent truth always reminds me of the pictures in the children's magazine and workbook called *Highlights*, in my pediatrician's office when I was a young boy. In these pictures, you were to find the parrot or the lion or the boat or whatever it was hidden in the line-drawn picture. However, if you didn't know what a parrot or lion or a boat looked like, how could you possibly recognize any of them in the drawing even when they were there in front of your face? How much of the truth of who we are can we not see? How much do we refuse to see or do we deny even when it is right in front of us?

The inability or refusal to see the shadow elements of ourselves is in itself an illness as is our reluctance to integrate those elements into the fullness of who we are and then live that fullness authentically. When we chose to live authentically, we dance in the light of our own revelation of ourselves; we dance in the truth of our own life story. When we dance in the light this way, our shadow also dances with us. We cannot dance in the light and not cast a shadow. The brighter the light, the greater and more distinct our shadow becomes. The more we dance, the more we see of our shadow and the more it is seen by others. On the contrary, the more we try to hide our shadow, the less we dance and the less we see of the light. Hence, to be who we were born to be in our fullest and to allow ourselves to be truly *seen* in the light of our own nakedness and vulnerability, in the light of our authenticity, requires the greatest courage and humility. Every intimate story of healing I have ever heard has been told to me by a heroic dancer.

Our life story is the key to who we are and the pages of our story that are most painful to us and not easily shared are the ones that are also most honest and descriptive of ourselves. These are the pages that show us in our nakedness and reveal our shadow elements and woundings. For our healing to begin, our life story must be told in its fullness and authenticity. And then, it must be heard. It must be witnessed and astutely and compassionately considered without judgment by another. We are *known* by our life stories. In the true telling of our story we inform the world of our struggles and the essential nature of our own existence because we are *seen* in our nakedness and our life is *witnessed* in its authenticity. In ironic contrast, when we truly *listen* to another's life story, when we see that person in their nakedness and toiling, we may be surprised to discover who we find there. We may find ourselves hiding between the lines of that other person's story and toiling in the lessons of their labors. For in truth, we are all one. We are all on the same transformational journey. We share in the same struggles this journey of life presents us as we navigate through the twists and turns of its fate and destiny. As we are witnessed by another, so do we witness. As we inform the world of our own existence, so do we inform the world of its own existence.

Our Story

All we have is our story. It is the only thing we can call our own. It is the only thing, when all is said and done, that will eternally be ours and ours alone. It will forever define us. Each one of us is a proper noun of life's existence while our story is the living verb and preposition of that existence in this specific time and place. Our story will never be told again in the particular way it has been told. It will never be lived by us again in the particular way it has been lived. Because of this, our life's story is sacred as is every living being's life story. Every life story is a living actuality of the self that experiences it and so each one of our life stories is a dynamic living expression of the "I" that lives it.

THIS NIGHT

This night;
  this
    deep,
    still,
    dark
    ocean
of a night;

This endless repository of
memory and dream
calls out to me . . .
screams
to me
with a vengeance
to remember.

I pretend to hear . . .
pretend to listen . . .
pretend to know.

But what do I know?

I know nothing,
I know only
this life.

All I can hear is
the voice of its existence . . .
the incessant pounding of this single heart
and
the persistent rhythm of this sequential breath
that keeps it all alive.

And then . . .
then
I remember
the one salient point of it all:

Even this shall pass.

© P. Donovan, 2007

As we live our story, it eventually becomes a revelation of itself. As it unfolds through time it becomes the defining benchmark of our identity, the defining proof of who we are and who we have been. As Jesus declared in Matthew 7.20, "By their fruits ye shall know them." Our life story is the story of our fruit. It is the historical accounting of the choices we have made, the actions we have taken, and the consequences to which we had to respond due to those choices and actions. These choices and their consequences are the true determinants of our identity. They are the fruit of our tree and our fruit is all we have to inform the world and ourselves of who we are.

Choosing to Choose

In biological systems, the identity of every living organism is revealed by three key characteristics: *structure, pattern of organization* and *process*. Each one of these characteristics is intertwined within and dependent upon the other two. The *structure* and *pattern of organization* of an organism (like our faces, body structures, and the patterns of living) are outcomes of the *process*. They are a result of the dynamic, evolutionary responses made by an organism in reaction to the various external and internal stimuli and influences encountered by that organism over time. *Process* is the history of changes resulting from those influences. In other words, *process* is the life story of an organism's existence. It is the verb and preposition of the organism's life story.

In the *process* of living our lives we, as a living organism, create the history of changes that occur to our *structure* and *pattern of organization*. We shape and form the *structure* and *pattern of organization* of who we are and what we become by the way in which we choose to live our lives . . . by the way we tell our story. In turn, our *structure* and *pattern of organization* (our facial features, height, physical capabilities, lifestyle, type of work, home environment, etc.) further influence and inform our story, and so on. We are formed and shaped on the anvil of time by the outcomes of our own choices. The history of our choices is written in the pages of our story. In short, we become who we choose to be and live the story we choose to tell with the functional word here being "choose."

Choice can only be exercised in the light of consciousness and only through the experience of differences, engendered by the perception of duality and separateness, can there be the possibility of choice. We can choose only because we are conscious, self-aware beings, cognizant of the "differences engendered by our separateness." We can choose also because we can imagine. We have developed the wonderful gift of imagination and because of that gift; we can imagine the myriad of potential outcomes of the numerous possibilities associated with each of our choices. Further, we can imagine those potentialities because of our experience of past choices and their resultant consequences. We can also imagine what the outcome possibilities to our choices might be through the historical stories of other people's lives and the consequences they experienced as a result of their choices. One thing for sure though, no matter how well we can imagine a possible outcome to a choice we make, there is never any certainty it will ever happen that way. That is the risk we take in making a choice. All choice is laced with uncertainty and risk.

We always exercise choice through "uncertainty" and "risk." Why through uncertainty? Because the consequences of any choice are never completely knowable just as the ending of our story is never completely knowable. Uncertainties and probabilities are woven into the fabric of the universe. As Heisenberg's "uncertainty principle" tells us, predetermined outcomes to any choice are nonexistent because all of the factors influencing a particular event at any one moment in time and space and all of the factors influencing those factors, *ad infinitum* can never be known. Why risk? Because risk is always looming in every choice we make. Every choice requires, to some degree, a loss of something known and familiar to make room for the birth of something new and not quite so familiar. Because of uncertainty, we can never be sure the loss of what we are losing is worth the value of what we are gaining. The only way to know anything for sure is to choose.

By choosing, we become an "I" and transform the quantum, non-local world of probabilities and potentialities into the materialized, local-world of our subjective reality. Our wave form of potentiality collapses and becomes solidified into the particle form of our material reality. By choosing, we risk the familiar and safe for the unfamiliar and unknown risky possibilities. By continuously choosing we are continuously creating; continuously growing, evolving, and self-affirming. This is what life is and what it does! Life is continuous creation. We write our life story through this directive of continuous creation and we do it following the plot of life's self-realization through self-affirmation. By our choices we are known. Choice is the chisel with which we sculpt and shape the reality of our existence, the reality of who and what we are. Life evolves and unfolds to become self-aware and realize its full potential and identity, through the continuous action of choice and the ever-present risk of pain and nonbeing associated with the outcomes of that choice. As the saying goes, "We make the bed we lie in."

As we live our lives, the history of our choices made through our lives, our "process," reveals the schematic theme of our existence; the schema of who we are and the theme of why we are here. If we do not examine this schematic theme daily, we will be unable to fully answer for ourselves the essential and fundamental questions of identity and purpose ("Who am I?" and "Why am I here?") because these questions remain unanswered in the "unexamined life." To "Above all, know thyself," we must answer these vital questions. We must examine our life daily. We must follow the way of its twists and turns of fate and destiny. We must inquire about the entrances and exits of all its many diverse characters: How long did they stay? Why did they come and why did they leave? We must consider the numerous intimate transactions of relational exchange into which we were seduced or seduced another in the name of love. Most certainly we must be watchful for the shadow that dances with us behind the footsteps of our conscious choreography.

References

1. Donovan, P & Joinerbey H: *The Face of Consciousness.* Lucky Press, 2006
2. Donovan, P: *This Night.* © P. Donovan, 2011

Chapter Four

Spaces

"The soul is wise and subtle; it recognizes that
unity fosters belonging. The soul adores unity.
What you separate, the soul joins."
(*John O'Donohue, Anam Cara:*
A Book of Celtic Wisdom, 1997)

"Your sacred space is where you can find
yourself again and again."
(*Joseph Campbell*)

The Space Between

There is a space between everything. In this three
dimensional reality of materialized particles, we
experience our self as a "thing." We are a person in a
world of separate "things" with spaces between us and between
everything. We are proper nouns in a world of nouns defined by
the space between us just as much as we are defined by the thing
we are and the space we occupy. The rhythm of our heartbeat
is defined just as much by the space between its beats as it is
by the beats themselves. The rhythm and melody of a song is
distinguished by the spacing of its notes on the musical score
just as much as it is by the notes themselves. It is the spaces that
determine how the song is played. In our lives, it is the spaces also,
that determine how our life is lived.

The spaces between us, between the events of our lives, the people we love, and the decisions we make dictate the rhythm and cadence of our life just as they do the rhythm and melody of a song. How often is it that we reference our lives by the spaces between meaningful events: "It was three years ago when we last saw each other." "We were married sixty two years ago today." "My mother died five years ago." and so forth. We celebrate in these spaces and we grieve in them. We are born in these spaces and we die in them. Most importantly, we live in them; we continuously create and become who we were born to be in them. They are not empty spaces.

The spaces between us and our world of things are filled with something otherworldly. They are filled with something sensual and wild; something not seen, only felt, intuited and experienced. They are filled with the spatial field potential of faith; "the substance of things hoped for and the evidence of things not seen," as defined in Hebrews 11:1. This field potential between us and the world around us is pregnant with the possibilities, potentialities and probabilities of our actions and choices. It influences and conditions the spaces between us in such a way that every "thing," from the smallest of subatomic particles to you and me and the greatest of celestial bodies, feels its influence and responds to its conditional dictates.

Although it occupies our spaces, this field of faith isn't a "thing." It influences the things within its space and directs the ordering of change. According to Rupert Sheldrake, Ph.D., proponent of the theory of morphic resonance, "Although energy can be regarded as the cause of change, the ordering of change depends on the spatial structure of the fields. These structures have physical effects, but they are not in themselves a type of energy; they act as 'geometrical' or spatial causes."[1]

In other words, in a world of nouns and proper nouns, the space between us and everything else is filled with a relational and probability matrix of prepositions, verbs and adverbs. Therefore, as proper nouns, we are differentiated and qualified by the prepositional and verb-like dictates of this relational matrix and its spatial conditioning. We are defined and given meaning by the space between us. We are given agency, direction, placement, timing, possession, and purpose by its prepositional attributes. By its verb and adverb-like properties, we are given action and our quality of being. Most importantly, however, we become something more than ourselves alone in this space because here is where the external world of "the other" is let in and embraced by us to be sensually experienced into our own subjective, internal reality of "self." It is here where we enter into relationship.

The Soul Adores Unity

All the spaces between us and the world around us are spaces of relationship. In these spaces we become more than who we are alone. We interact with the outside world to become a lover, a friend, a husband or a wife, a father or a mother, a brother or a sister, and so forth. On the darker side, in these spaces we can also become a killer, a thief, a victim, or someone we may not like. As we activate the prepositional or verbal phrasing of this spatial field matrix of potentialities, we clarify and define ourselves by the fruit of our actions and choices. We must be careful in these spaces. We do not dance alone here.

In the spaces between us we dance with others. Therefore, with whom we choose to dance and how we choose to dance with them determines what we become. Are you a lover or are you a thief? We must choose wisely with whom we fill our spaces and which prepositions and verbs we want to define us in the matrices of our spaces. If we fill them with love, we will be loved and dance with lovers. If we fill them with fear, we will be fearful and dance with adversaries, liars and thieves to the tune of victimization and resentment. If we must dance with adversaries, it is important we choose only worthy ones who can reveal our deficits and challenge our possibilities. This way we can grow.

I think of every space between us as being a "doorway to the kingdom of God," a doorway to the inside of the inside where the Divine Spirit that dwells in each one of us has her abode. Spirit resides in the spaces between us as the guiding and ordering field of probabilities and continuous creation. I see the space between everything as the birthplace of all creation, as the field matrix from which every particle relationship in the universe is conceived, nurtured and born into being. I cannot imagine the Divine Spirit as a noun or a thing. I imagine Divine Spirit as relational; as a state of being and relating that, like a spatial field potential of probabilities, orders the relationships and directs the conditions of being for all of us and for everything throughout the universe. Simply put, the Divine Spirit is and has Her abode within the space between everything. She is the embodiment of relationship.

Where "two or more are gathered" in the name of relationship, there too is Divine Spirit. When there are two or more of us gathered together there are always spaces between us. In these spaces, Spirit resides. Here, in these spaces, we are seen and witnessed by those present and by Divine Spirit. We are witnessed in the action and quality of our being and, as we are witnessed, we in turn witness others. In these spaces, we dance the great dance of relationship where the creative hand of intimacy and love, of Divine Spirit works its artistic magic to form us into something greater than ourselves. That "something" that is more

45

than ourselves is what the Jewish mystic and philosopher Martin Buber, refers to as "Thou."

I and Thou

As we experience ourselves as a proper noun, we experience ourselves as an "I" separate from the other "Is" and "its" of the world. We are separated by the space between us. However, when that space is filled with relationship, when we are seen in that space and become known in it, we are no longer an "it." We are no longer alone. We become something more than an "it" or an "I." We become a "somebody," somebody "known" to someone other than our self. We are then transformed from the limited individual I consciousness of separateness into the inclusive Thou consciousness of relationship: a more universal and contextual consciousness of being. As Martin Buber, writes in his book, *I and Thou*: "The person who emerges from the act of pure relation that so involves his being has now in his being something more that has grown in him, of which he did not know before . . . ."[2]

That "something more" that grows in us is the realization of ourselves as a part of something greater than ourselves alone. We realize ourselves as a part of a marriage, a family, a community, a race, or as a part of life itself. When we enter into relationship with another, we take part in an act of unification and true individual self-affirmation. As we become I we recognize our beingness in and identity with something more than I. We recognize ourselves as being part of the greater whole, a holon of a greater holon. As Buber states, "The primary word I-Thou can be spoken only with the whole being. Concentration and fusion into the whole being can never take place through my agency alone, nor can it ever take place without me. I become through my relationship to the Thou; as I become I, I say Thou."[3]

When we enter into relationship with compassion and love, when we fill our spaces with them, we influence the spatial field of the Divine Spirit with that compassion and love. The resulting Thou we become is transformational, boundless, and godlike. It nourishes and sustains us, guides and protects us on our life's journey to become all that we were born to be. Even something more happens when we fill our spaces with compassion and love. We then transform all those with whom we dance into something more than they are. The ugly become beautiful, the weak become strong, the threatening become reassuring, and we free them to be all that they were born to be. As Buber further writes, "In the eyes of him who takes his stand in love, and gazes out of it, men are cut free from their entanglement in bustling activity. Good people and evil, wise and foolish, beautiful and ugly, become successively real to him; that is, set free they step forth in their singleness and confront him as "Thou."[4]

Countless people have become "successively real" to me over the many years of my medical practice. When I could be present for them and could "take my stand in love and gaze out of it" at their stories of struggle and pain, at their stories of illness and healing, they "stepped forth in their singleness" and "confronted me as Thou." I cannot describe to you thoroughly enough here what that has meant to me, what it has given me and how it has changed me. It has been an honor and yet a heavy weight to bare, a weight like so many other care givers and people who take their stand in love bare when they witness the stories of another. We become the keepers of the stories we are told and their weight is what we carry until we die. There is a saying, "We die two deaths: The death when we pass from this plane of existence and a second death when the last person on earth who carries and knows our story dies."

The Space Inside

There is a space inside of us. We call it the human soul. In it there is a mirror. This mirror reflects into the spaces outside of us all that we are of soul inside. Our bodies are a reflection from this mirror. They are the materialized expression of our soul as it is reflected into the spatial field of form. Our soul desperately longs for an outer expression of itself. As John O'Donohue writes, "All our inner life and intimacy of soul longs to find an outer mirror. It longs for a form in which it can be seen, felt, and touched."[5] Our soul longs for the intimacy of relationship so that it can be seen, felt, and touched. It longs to be known.

Our soul did not create itself. It was born from the space of Divine Spirit to become the space we occupy as self. This is essentially a Platonic and Neoplatonic concept. As the ancient Greek philosopher Plotinus instructs: from the One there is the Intelligence, there is Soul, from which comes souls. We are our soul and from this space of soul we reflect our inner presence into the outer world of form to become known. Our bodies occupy the space of our soul. They interpret the presence of our soul into the facial expressions and physical actualization of its essence. Sometimes our faces occupy the greatest presence of our soul. In some people, the story of their soul is most clearly written in the lines and structure of their faces. In others, it is written more clearly in their bodies and the way in which they carry themselves and act. Yet, in still others, their soul story is most clearly told in their speech, their voice and the words and phraseologies they choose to describe their lives and the livers of others. The most predominant and clearest presence of our soul, however, is appreciated most commonly in our eyes. It is said our eyes are the windows of our soul. Actually, they are the windows through which we can see the space of our soul. When someone says, "His or her eyes are so deep." It is because the space of that person's soul is so deep. I find the more life experience we have had, the more transformational changes we have struggled and toiled through, the deeper and more expansive the space of our soul becomes.

Wisdom is a result of the deeper and more expansive space of our soul. With wisdom, we see the wholeness and "bigger picture" of a situation because we can accommodate more of it in our soul space. Love also deepens our soul space. Love is expansive and inclusive. It makes room in our soul for the people and things we love. When we love, we let what it is we love into our space. The more we love, the more we let into our space and so, the bigger our inner space becomes. There are things that limit and shrink our soul space, however. Of these things, fear is the biggest. Fear is restrictive and exclusive. It retracts and shrinks away from that which it fears and so, it restricts our soul space. We have less room for anything when we fill our soul space with fear; less room for people, family, friends, ideas, even facts when they are presented to us. When fear shrinks our soul space small enough, we perceive everything as a threat and we strike out at everything with a vengeance to save our soul. We end up saving nothing while our soul eventually shrivels up into nothingness as it starves itself of the very nourishment it needs to survive.

We are the spaces we occupy and we are born of Divinity. We are known through the spaces between us. How we are known is dependent on how we dance and with whom we dance in these spaces. Sometimes the dance is painful and not easy and other times it is ecstatic. As Theodore Roosevelt proclaimed:

"The credit belongs to the person who is actually in the arena; whose face is marred by sweat and blood; who strives valiantly; who errors and comes short again because there is no effort without error and shortcoming; who knows the great enthusiasms, the great devotion, spends himself in a worthy cause; who at best knows in the end the triumph of high achievement; and who at worst, if he fails, at least fails while daring greatly so that his place will never be with those cold and timid souls who have never tasted victory or defeat."[6]

References

1. Sheldrake R: *A New Science of Life*. Rochester, VT: Park Street Press, 1995; 60
2. Buber, M: *I and Thou*. New York: Scribner's Sons, 1958; 109
3. Ibid. 11
4. Ibid. 15
5. O'Donohue, J: *Anam Cara: A Book of Celtic Wisdom*. New York: HarperCollins, 1997; 47
6. Theodore Roosevelt quotes, American 26th U.S. President, 1901-09 (1858-1919)

Chapter Five

The Burning Ground

"And I take you down to the burning ground
And you change me up and you turned it around."
(From the song, "The Burning Ground" by Van Morrison, 1997.)

The Fire of Profound Relating

The burning ground is a place of purification. It is the ground in the space between us where we go to hash out our differences and come to an understanding. Every relationship has its burning ground; that place where we go with another in our honesty and authenticity to, as Van Morrison sings, "change things up" and "turn them around." As with any relationship, this is not an easy place to be. It is difficult and very uncomfortable to say the least. We are naked here and confront the shadows of ourselves and others here as we find ourselves dancing around relationship's fire of intrapersonal conflicts and ego agendas. As we dance, we project our shadows in the light of this fire and we dance with them so that we might turn them around and become a Thou.

The burning ground is a place of hard work and sweat and profound relating. It is no place for pleasantries or "political correctness." Such facades are quickly charred and seared to a blackened flesh by the heat of this fire's intimacy, candor and directness. We cannot hide or be idle here either. This is not a place for cowards or wimps. We must be fully present and accessible.

We can't enter this ground with cell phones and emails and we can't text our way in or out. We are forced to work hard on this often times battle ground of light and shadow if we are to remain in the dance. We are expected to fight, negotiate, surrender, leave or transform into something more here. It is always our choice. But, there are no other options for us here.

The burning ground is also a place of ashes. We burn things here if and when we have the courage and humility to dump them on this purifying fire and watch them turn to ashes and smoke. We burn our dead here; our dead thoughts, feelings, beliefs, relationships, and ways of living and relating that no longer serve us in a productive and life-affirming way. They are burned in the transformational and self-reflective flames of relationship's fire as we struggle to become something more than our selves yet not lose our selves in the process. We also burn our ego here as it is a collector of dead things. Ego hoards the old and familiar. It hoards them even after their days of utility have long past. There is no security in old and dead things to be had here if we are to thrive. There is only opportunity for growth and newness arising from the smoke and ashes of their sacrifice.

The burning ground is a place of phoenix magic and hero stories. When we enter this sacred ground of purification with humility and openness, in our authenticity and realness, people "step forth in their singleness and confront us as Thou." In that confrontation, we see each other in the light of this fire's heat. In that light of profound relating, all is revealed to each other. Stories are shared and faces become more actual and familiar while shadows become more frightening and monstrous. Our task in this place is to understand what monsters in our selves need to be slain and then slay them, and what stories and faces need to be embraced and then embrace them. When we do this with love and humility, we "emerge from this act of pure relation that so involves our being, with something more." Where we entered as an "I", we now emerge as a "We" changed and transformed by the phoenix magic of real and profound relating.

The Monsters We Slay Are Always Our Own

When we leave our obsessive distraction and preoccupation with "things" for the ground of the spaces between them, life becomes more real and palpable. When we dialogue with voice instead of texting and hear the inflections of emotion while we gaze into the spaces of another's eyes with presence, we participate in the organic alchemy of life that transmutes the lead of our aloneness into the unifying gold of our profound relating. When we leave the safety of complacency and denial and *willingly* confront the shadow elements of our illness stories, new stories of heroes and healing emerge that will be remembered and told for lifetimes. The stories of defeat and failure created out of the shadow elements of our woundings and illness become the stories of our triumph and healing. I remember a saying from one of my mentors when I was younger: "Our lowest point of detriment can become our highest point of glory." Our lowest point of illness, therefore, can become our greatest point of healing.

Over the years of hearing so many stories of illness, I have come to experience the pathological themes of those stories as commonly rooted in a chronic neuroses blooming with feelings of fear, guilt, anxiety, depression, loneliness, and separateness. These distressing feelings and thoughts are the allegorical "demons," "dragons" and "monsters" of "the shadow world" often met by the mythological Heroes or Heroines along their perilous journey as told in so many of our cultural and mythic stories. The dragons and monsters we slay are always our own. Avoiding these denizens of our shadow world and triumphantly continuing our life's journey into healing is not a possibility for any of us. Here is where we are asked to risk our life so that we may find our life. In the transmutational act of slaying our shadow elements we slay ourselves; crucified, we are resurrected, dismembered we are then reborn. As the mythologist, Joseph Campbell instructs us in his book, *The Hero With A Thousand Faces*: "When our day has come for the victory of death, death closes in; there is nothing we can do, except be crucified and resurrected; dismembered totally and then reborn."[1]

Living authentically with emotional honesty while being present with others in the continuous act of profound relating allows us the opportunity to confront and slay these shadow demons of our illness stories. Living in this manner allows us to deeply acknowledge and experience our truest and often times most frightening feelings so they may reveal to us the source of our suffering and the solution to the riddle of our illness and struggle. This confrontation and acknowledgement has been referred to mystically as "going into the fires of initiation" with reference to the mythical phoenix and its transformational "ascent from the ashes." It is also mythologically represented by the hero's "entry into the cave," into the "dragon's lair" or the "witch's castle." It has also been represented by the hero's "crucifixion," "wounding," or "descent into the underworld" where he/she must die as a commoner so as to be resurrected as a hero/heroine. Scientifically, this act of dying to be reborn represents the evolutionary journey of life's continuous creation as it constantly evolves through chaos into ever increasing levels of new order and complexity, diversity, self-awareness, and self-affirmation.

I have come to understand illness as being the evidence of our struggle to defeat and transform the monsters of our shadow elements into the heroic deeds of our life's story. I see it as the evidence of our essential essence and nature of being struggling to affirm itself against the inertia, complacency and denial of unconscious, uncreative and instinctual living. As I said in chapter one, illness is the very process through which we are healed. Through the struggle of our illness we are reborn anew, we are made whole again. All healing, like all illness knows only one goal, to make us become whole.

The Act of Sacrifice is Organic

When we dance before the fire on the burning ground of light and shadow, we are expected to bring gifts for the fire. These gifts are the carcasses of the monsters we have slain by our introspective swords and self-affirming dance in this sacred space of profound relating. They stoke the fire and become the sacrificial smoke that rises to the Divine as the sweet incense of our prayer. It has been said, "All prayer must include an act of sacrifice." In this universe of action and reaction, of give and take, something must be lost so that something new can be gained. There is always a price to be paid for our healing, for our passage through chaos into new order. This has always been historically intuited by our ancestors. They understood the meaning and power of the sacrificial act in their daily lives because they lived so close to nature. They understood it as the price that had to be paid for new life because they were immersed daily in the cycles of birth, death, and rebirth. They knew, the act of sacrifice is organic.

Everywhere we look in the natural world around us, we witness the continual act of sacrifice, of new life emerging out of the death and disintegration of old life. I have watched for hours the last struggling moments of a salmon's life as it graciously surrendered its life to the inevitable beauty of its own continuous creation in a small forest pool miles away from the familiarity of the ocean's currents it new so well. In that very same forest, I have also seen the new cedar saplings sprouting from the decomposing stumps of an earlier life which had now become a sacrificial death providing for the emergence of new life. Life renews itself through the sacrifice of itself. As Tillich writes, "Self-affirmation is the affirmation of life and of the death which belongs to life."[2] Dying from one realm of existence in the cycle of life is tantamount to being born to another realm of existence, another level of consciousness or organizational complexity. This is how we grow. Our life, as we live it, derives much of its meaning and preciousness from its struggle through the unremitting occurrences of death. For us to continually grow and evolve we must continually die on some level. Something of the old must give way for something of the new.

> "If we must die, let it not be like hogs
> Hunted and penned in an inglorious spot,
> While round us bark the mad and hungry dogs,
> Making their mock at our accursèd lot.
> If we must die, O let us nobly die
> So that our precious blood may not be shed
> In vain; then even the monsters we defy
> Shall be constrained to honor us though dead!"[3]

Our sacrificial acts were never meant to be sacrifices of lambs, of children, or of each other. Each life is sovereign and that sovereignty is to be respected. The sacrifice we bring to the burning ground has always been meant to be one of our own, a sacrifice of our own egoic surrender. What of ego do we surrender to the fire? We surrender our shadow elements to the fire; those feelings, ideas, and beliefs that are no longer life-generating and life-affirming. Old patterns of fear, complacency, denial and resistance to life's transformative changes are sacrificed on the fire as they are discovered through our dance in the burning ground of profound relating. They are surrendered to make way for new patterns of self-actualization and self-affirmation, to make room for growth. If we want to drink new tea, we must be willing to empty our cup of the old tea.

To sacrifice is to offer, give up or surrender something prized or desirable for the sake of something considered as having a higher or more pressing claim. The surrendering of our egoic illusion of separateness and its resultant neuroses and feelings of fear, aloneness, and isolation is the hero's gift that brings us new life. This gift is not an easy gift for any of us to relinquish even with its promise of new life. Most of us are dragged into this proposition by the seat of our pants, kicking and screaming. We are commonly more comfortable with the devils we know. Bit by bit, however, we slowly acquiesce to the sacrificial summons of the dance under the directive of life's self-affirming mandate. Eventually our sacrifices turn us away from egocentric and selfish living and we step forth in our realness to become *Thou*. As John Briggs and David Peat describe in their book, *Seven Life Lessons of Chaos*, "In each moment, we have the opportunity to die psychologically by letting go of prejudices, mechanical habits, isolation, precious ego, images of self and world, and conceptions of the past and future. In this way, we set in motion the possibility of a creative, self-organizing perception that puts us in touch with the magic that gave us birth."[4]

Now, there is a poignant question begged here. "What must die in me? What prejudices, mechanical habits, feelings of isolation, precious ego illusions, images of self and world, and conceptions of the past and future must I throw into the sacrificial fire of transformation to put me in touch with the magic that gave me birth?" I can't answer these questions for you. Only you can answer them for yourself. However, those with whom you have danced and those with whom you continue to dance are the best qualified to help you. They have seen your shadow dancer dancing behind you in the light of relationship's fire and you have seen theirs. Parents, siblings, lovers, friends, and even adversaries may know at least some of the answers to this question. Through them, you may find the answers to these following questions useful: Why do you love me? Why did you leave me? Why do I love you? Why did I leave you? What irritates me about you? What irritates you about me? What do I admire about you? What do you admire about me?

We can learn much by the friends we keep and the adversaries we create. Each one is our teacher revealing to us the next step in our dance and what new gift we can bring to the fire. Each one enters and exits our life or stays according to a rhythm, a cadence set lifetimes ago by the tempo of our dance and the choices of our lives. We would do well to be present with each one of these dance partners so that we may clearly hear their direction as they offer to us their guidance through the struggles of our fated illnesses and limitations. What they offer us may be lead or it may be gold. We choose! The direction is ours to take, or not.

Smoke and Mirrors

We must choose well what gifts we place upon the fire. It is easy to become confused by the ego agendas of the other dancers as well as our own. The structure and function of our ego is one of self-protection and survival. Just the mention of sacrifice or death of any kind, even when it means greater growth and self-actualization, causes our ego to jump into hyper-mode. Neurosis can arise from this hyper-mode when we are too "sensitive" and fully open to the world around us, especially if our boundaries of self are weak or unclear. Our ego will do all it can to protect us and make sure we survive even into the realm of ridiculousness. When this occurs, we may become anxiety-laden and paralyzed by fears emerging in us about all sorts of nonthreatening things and situations. Or, we may become hypersensitive and allergic to common, nonthreatening substances in our environments and react to them violently to assure us we avoid them.

This egoic hyper-mode can also push us into greed, fraud, genocide, and war, when all we experience of self is the "limited self" or "unawakened self." This is the self of eat, sleep, procreate, and the maintenance of personal pleasure and power. This is the self that is minimally aware of anything or anyone else in the world outside of its own egocentric reality. Those of us living in this limited experience of selfness haven't yet or are not yet able to step into the burning ground of profound relating and be fully present there for the dance and the fire. It is difficult for any of us living in this limited reality of self to "step forth in our realness as *I* and say *Thou*," thereby realizing our beingness in something greater than our self, alone. Those of us in this reality of self are not yet able to conceive of ourselves as belonging to a Greater Self of inclusiveness and unity; unable to perceive our self as an individual expression of the Divine Spirit. As a result of this, we then often live in a more fear-based exclusivistic existence as opposed to an existence that is more inclusive and compassion-based. In this fear-based existence of the limited self, we see most everything and everyone as a threat to us and avoid them by either controlling them or eliminating them.

Our ego mind is commonly associated with the trickster or the fool in our cultural mythologies. Commonly we see it played by the coyote or crow in Native American folk tales. Focused on self-preservation, our ego will do all it can to trick us into staying safe and secure. Not that this is a bad thing. But, when it constrains our growth and self-affirming ability to be all that we were born to be, it becomes entropic and paralyzing. We can get so preoccupied with our safety and security that we limit our experience of life to one of ennui and stagnation. The irony here is we end up dying anyway. We just die a slower death, a long drawn out entropic death couched in front of our TVs and iPhones rarely dancing on that sacred ground of profound relatedness. We end up sacrificing much in this kind of death. There are no great, heroic stories here. No dragons or monsters slain and too few people to carry our story for us when we die; what little story we have to tell.

Our intellect is the home of our ego while our heart is the home of our soul. When we dance on sacred ground, we must dance with our hearts so that we are assured we are dancing with soul; dancing with authenticity, humility, and integrity. If we dance with our intellect, we will dance with the trickster. We may then be easily fooled into thinking the things we are called to place on the sacrificial fire are of value to our transformative growth when all they are, are smoke and mirrors. Our ego does not surrender easily that which has given us value, safety, pleasure, and comfort in the past. It diligently refuses to give up the survival, pleasure, and comfort mechanisms that worked for us even though they have long passed served their purpose. If what our heart decides to throw upon the sacrificial fire is of value to our ego, our ego will not be willing to let go of it easily. Our ego will work hard to convince us through intellectual reasoning and rationalization, something else of lesser value would be more appropriate. The key to seeing through this smoke and mirror game is in how loudly and vehemently our ego protests. To quote Shakespeare (with a little adaptation) from Hamlet, Act III, Scene II: "Thee [ego] doth protest too much, methinks."

There are many times when our heart must just say no to our ego's intellectual rationalizations to promote its self-protective and self-gratifying agendas. Our intellect, at the biding of ego, can rationalize anything for the benefit and preservation of our ego-comforts, control and security. It can even rationalize murder, war and genocide as we can too easily witness in the history of our world and in our daily news. I have heard it said by many wise persons, "The ego rationalizes while the heart knows." I have to agree with this, from my experience. What our heart knows is of the soul and what is of the soul is Divine. The heart's knowing is intuitive and originates from the *Thou* experience of inclusion and wholeness. It originates from "the magic that gave us birth."

I have found truth to be known by the heart. It is felt and experienced deep within that space inside of us. Our heart has sensitivity to truth. It resonates with truth when it is in the presence of truth. Intellect doesn't feel truth as the heart does. It tries instead to rationalize truth to accommodate a particular situation or moment in time. We can rationalize just about anything we want to believe whether it is true or not, factual or not. Belief does not require truth. Truth has always presented itself to me as something ageless, constant, and dependable that describes reality in some way. I think of it as a fundamental principle underlying reality. It is commonly defined as "the property of being in accord with fact or reality" or as "a transcendent fundamental or spiritual reality." Therefore, when we know a truth we are empowered by it because we are then rooted in the fact and reality of that truth. We can argue many beliefs even our belief in truth, but truth, in itself, has little argument.

Over the years of guiding my patients through their healing process, I have found their beliefs to be the greatest source of resistance to their healing. In fact, their beliefs frequently are the cause of their illness. For all of us, beliefs can get in our way more than they can help us when it comes to our healing process and our personal growth. As egoic constructs to assure our safety and security, our beliefs can hold us prisoner to prejudices, mechanical habits, feelings of isolation, precious ego illusions, images of self and world, and conceptions of the past and future that no longer facilitate our growth or further our self-actualization. They do, however, keep us safe and secure in old, redundant and familiar habits and patterns of living even when our beliefs have little to no evidence of fact or reality to support them. When we are dancing on the burning ground of sacred space and it comes time for us to gift the fire for our healing, we can be sure of this: The gift we sacrifice to the fire will be something of our own; our heart will know what that is; our ego will diligently protest it and; it will be something of our belief.

Some people may be curious here about faith and may ask the question, "How does faith play into this idea of belief and knowing?" I like to think of faith as a knowing based on some evidence of reality and substance of fact. Even the Bible defines faith as requiring some substance of fact and evidence of reality as it states, ". . . faith is the *substance of things* hoped for, the *evidence of things not seen*." (Hebrews 11:1) My favorite definition of faith was given to me by one of my mentors when I was younger. Ruth liked to say, "Faith is acting as if it is already done." Healing is acting as if it is already done. Once we sacrifice those elements of ourselves that have resisted our healing and our transformational growth, we must proceed from the fire and the dance knowing and acting as if our healing is already done and our transformation has already taken place.

References

1. Campbell J: *The Hero With A Thousand Faces. Princeton University Press*, 1973
2. Tillich P: *The Courage To Be.* 1952, 28
3. From the poem by Claude McKay: *If We Must Die.* First published,1919
4. Briggs J and Peat D: *Seven Life Lessons of Chaos.* Harper Collins, NY, 1999; 30

Chapter Six

Fear and the Old Prayer

"Our deepest fear is not that we are inadequate. Our
deepest fear is that we are powerful beyond measure. It
is our light, not our darkness that most frightens us."
(*Marianne Williamson, Return to Love: Reflections
on the Principles of "A Course in Miracles"*)

"Most people do not really want freedom,
because freedom involves responsibility, and most
people are frightened of responsibility."
(*Sigmund Freud, Civilization and Its Discontents*)

"A man that flies from his fear may find that
he has only taken a short cut to meet it."
(*J.R.R. Tolkien, The Children of Húrin*)

The Old F—k You Prayer

Just as I have come to realize the utility of illness in the healing process, I have come to appreciate fear as a function of courage. Courage can only be realized in the presence of fear. Upon asking if a man can still be brave if he is afraid, Bran is told by his father, in George R.R. Martin's, *A Game of Thrones*, "That is the only time a man can be brave!" Our bravery and courage to continue forward through fear is a function of our will. Fear strengthens our will; clarifies our will. It teaches us how precious and dear life is to us and how precious and dear we

64

are to ourselves. Fear, when we conquer it and move through it, is a functional aspect of will. However, when we are caught in it, when fear controls us, it becomes a dysfunctional form of will. When this happens, it drags us into an entropic paralysis where living becomes a greater threat to us than dying. I have watched too many of my patients allow themselves to be dragged into this place of paralysis by fear to the point where they unconsciously choose death rather than courageously face living.

Now I can certainly understand how the unremitting stresses of our lives can ware on us over time. Some of the many life stories I have heard over these years have been heartrending and distressing enough just to have heard and witnessed more or less to have been lived. As I am writing this very paragraph, I am disturbed by a phone call from one of my good colleagues and past students. After nearly two years of going through a father's hell with his son's cancer, his young son and only child, was just found to have another recurrence of his high-risk neuroblastoma. Few children survive these high-risk forms. I am a father; I can only imagine his struggle, his pain, and his feelings of helplessness and guilt. We talked about this for a while. Life, and its many struggles, can be too much to bear at times for many of us. At those times it feels easier to "tap the mat" and give up the fight, than it does to continue onward. The fear of living through more pain and yet another struggle can sometimes be more acutely threatening to us than the fear of death itself. This is the time the old "f—k you" prayer, as clarified for me by an elderly Irish priest, comes in handy.

In 2007, I was experiencing a lot of grief and emotional pain working through a divorce, a move, caring for my ill and deteriorating parents as well as my children, and managing a medical practice while also teaching at the university. After slamming the trunk of my car on my head (forgetting the bike rack was still on it) and knocking myself out on my driveway in the pouring rain one frustrating November evening, I decided I had enough and needed to get away for a while and go to Ireland. I rented a small cottage in a little village outside of Gendalough. This cottage happened to be near to the only church in this village. One Sunday, trying to escape the monotonous and incessant pounding of the Irish rain on the "tin" roof of my cottage, I went driving the Irish roads. I drove them like the angry and crazy Irishman I was at the time, swearing at myself and the Universe for the seemingly endless torment of struggle I had been experiencing. Anyone who has driven the Irish country roads knows how bad of an idea this was. After going over a small bridge and realizing my tires weren't touching the road due to my speed, I decided it was time to get back to the cottage and take a deep breath.

As I approached the cottage well after ten o'clock in the evening, I noticed a light on in the church rectory. Father Kevin was still up. Now I had never meant Father Kevin but I knew I needed to talk to someone of his ilk so that I might be able to clarify some choices I had to make. I knocked at Father Kevin's door and he greeted me with a smile and his priestly collar undone and invited me in. "Tea, my son?" "Yes, sure Father. That would be great," I replied. We began to talk. In the midst of our conversation, Father Kevin asked me if I had been praying. I told him, "Yes Father. I have been praying but you might not approve of the delivery or style of my prayer." "How have ya been prayin' now, my son?" he asked. I told him the best I could do as a prayer was to punch the steering wheel repeatedly of the car as I was driving and shout at God saying, "F—k you! F—k you! F—k you!" Well, with that said Father Kevin promptly stood up, walked to the cabinet next to us, pulled out a small bottle of fine Irish whiskey and poured a generous shot into each of our cups of tea and sat down. Then he said, with the most compassionate and understanding sparkle in his eye, "Ah yes, the old f—k you prayer. I know it well." We talked long that good night, well into the early morning hours.

THE SHADOW OF LIGHT

I came to Ireland to be alone again in some very powerful places . . . to realize again the deep Celtic heart of this land . . . of my heart and the heart of my father(s). I came to Ireland to heal a broken heart and face down the "beasts" of my own shadow and the shadow of my father(s). It was a powerful experience facing them both at the same time alone in the land of their origin . . . in the dark, heavy, melancholy and unremitting rain and dampness of this proud yet so deeply wounded place. Driven by my personal inquisition and the genetic beasts of my inner narrative, I found myself at the rectory door of an Irish priest and the conversation of a lifetime. I then began to understand the darkness . . . its power to transform things and invite the light . . . no, its power to demand of the light its presence; demand the light TO BE. Light emerges from the darkness . . . always overcomes yet contains the darkness within itself. This is the blood-truth of the Celtic soul. This is the blood-truth of life.

P. Donovan, Dublin, 2007

I learned something very valuable that night from Father Kevin. When we are faced with the fear and frustration of living due to the incessant and overwhelming torment of our struggle; when we find ourselves thinking more about dying than we are about living, it is time for "the old f—k you prayer" and it's alright. It's OK to be angry and fed up with ourselves and the life situation we find ourselves in. It is alright to say, "F—k you!" to the world and to ourselves when we have had enough. It can even be therapeutic to say "Fuck you!" to The Divine and let The Divine know we are at the end of our resources. It is out of this frustration and anger, change and healing finally emerges. The key here, however, is change. We must then do something to change our situation and not allow ourselves to be a victim of it any longer. That something most likely will require three things:

1) Identifying, facing and overcoming the deep, secret fear that is at the source of our struggle and illness;

2) Thinking creatively so that what we chose to do isn't the same thing we've been doing leading us to the same outcomes repeatedly. To continue to do the same thing and expect a different outcome is hopeless if not to say ridiculous.

3) Asking for help from our own "Father Kevin." That could be anyone we respect, professional or personal, who can go to the burning ground with us and be present for our story. They then can act as a sounding board outside the box and reflect back to us our struggle with new perspectives we could not see before. A trained healthcare provider can also be invaluable here.

The Secret Fear

Many of us have had and may still have a fear of the dark. It is theorized by most schools of psychology, our fear of the dark arises from our fear of the unknown and the possibility of unseen dangers lurking in the depth of the darkness threatening our survival. This is certainly an important component of the fear of the dark. However, I am going to suggest a theory here that is something completely different, one involving a primal fear that is rarely acknowledged or discussed. I suggest a more primal fear to be the *fear of our own Light*. When we are "in the dark," that darkness requires of us our Light that we may find our way. When our Light shines, we become aware of where we are and where we need to go on our once darkened, now enlightened path. As with healing requiring illness for its realization and fulfillment, and life requiring death for its renewal and regeneration, the manifestation and appearance of our own light requires the darkness for its expression. Light is not light, without the essential possibility and existential reality of darkness.

We all know dark places require light to reveal not only the unseen dangers hidden there but also the pathway leading us out. Light is power. It reveals and makes clear to us our pathway on our journey in this life and the dangers we need to avoid. If we are the one holding the flashlight in the dark forest at night with friends, it is WE who then have the power of discernment and clarity. To paraphrase psychologist and mythologist Eric Neumann, light is the symbol of consciousness and self-awareness. Only in that light can we know our way in the world.[1] From Neumann's perspective then, for us to manifest our light and illuminate our way through the dark places in our life, we need to be conscious and self-aware. I agree with Neumann. I think our light is revealed to us and illuminates our way when we live consciously in our authenticity. When we live creatively the fullness of who we are, accountable to and responsible for ourselves and our choices, we manifest our light to the world and the meaning of our life is then revealed to us in that light.

Oh, but even as I write this phrase, "accountable to and responsible for ourselves and our choices," something inside of me shutters with fear. Something in those words makes me draw back and reconsider. Why? Why is it, that not only me but nearly every one with whom I have known in my personal and professional experience retracts in some way from these words of accountability and responsibility? I have come to realize it is because of fear. What we truly fear about our light is the responsibility and accountability required of us and the freedom it generates when we live in the light of our truth. Freud informs us, "Most people do not really want freedom, because freedom involves responsibility, and most people are frightened of responsibility." Ego has no way out when we are responsible and accountable. It can't protect itself by projecting its failures or deficits on to someone or something else. It must be accountable to them and responsible for them and risk the judgment, criticism, or even punishment that may result.

Freedom is scary. I remember backpacking and hitchhiking around Ireland in 1971, when I was nineteen years old. It was just me, my backpack, and my guitar. I was fully accountable to and responsible for no one else but myself at the time. I had no "planned" destination and woke up every morning with the excitement of the new adventure the day would bring. I was free! It was one of the best times of my life, yet one of the most frightening. I was too young to know who I was then and too frightened to find out. So, I left Ireland and came home earlier than I planned after weeks of roaming the Irish countryside by myself discovering my freedom.

I find many of my patients in this same predicament regarding their illness. They are too limited in their knowledge of who they are and why they may be ill and too frightened to find out; frightened of the light of their own self-revelation and the freedom it allows them. Their fear restrains them and holds them back in illness; prevents them from realizing the story of their healing hidden in the story of their illness. Their story of healing calls them into accountability and offers them freedom. For many, this is too frightening. Instead, the proposition of death and illness is easier for them to handle then the riskier proposition of freedom and the self-revelation healing offers. They would rather remain in the dark.

I am now convinced the greatest actual obstacle to our healing is our fear of being well. Healing and wellness carry with them the promise of freedom and that promise can be frightening for many of us, especially if our illness works for us in some dysfunctional way. This fear is not easily revealed or discussed by us. When it is revealed to us, we will have to act on it. Therefore, it is kept in a secret unconscious place by our ego so that it won't be discovered and called out. When it is discovered, our ego protests loudly with intellectual rationalizations and excuses because it doesn't want to give up the habits of our illness easily even if they are self-destructive; it doesn't want to give up the security, comfort, pleasures, or control our illness offers us. This may be hard to understand for many people reading this. But I swear I have seen this many, many times with my patients suffering from chronic illness. This is especially true when their illness allows them some sort of dysfunctional control or is a result of unhealthy diets and life styles that give them pleasure. In such scenarios, our illness becomes the excuse for our failure to live fully and authentically.

I first got an eye-opening glimpse of this scenario many years ago when I was caring for a middle-aged woman with M.S. In a deep and probing conversation with her in my office, she told me her husband of twenty eight years had made some substantial changes since her illness with regards to their marriage. When I asked her how he had changed, she told me he was now coming home from work every night to take care of her instead of hanging out until late drinking with his men friends. He even made her dinner most nights now. Before her paralyzing illness, he wasn't coming home until after eight o'clock in the evening and gave her little attention. Now, she had all the attention from him she wanted and needed. In fact, with more probing questions on my part, I discovered she was actually able to control him with her illness. She used helplessness and guilt as her mechanisms of control. Through her illness, she was now able to get what she wanted from her husband. If she was to get well again, she would risk losing that attention from him and control of him. She settled instead for M.S. because it worked so well for her. Partial paralysis was a reasonable price to pay for his attention and she no longer had to openly deal with the interpersonal and personal problems that contributed to their marriage woes driving her husband away from home every night.

The choices we make regarding our fear of freedom; our fear of coming into our full power as an individual, are not commonly conscious choices. We don't usually plan out how we are going to avoid our fear of freedom and responsibility. We aren't even typically aware this fear exists because it hides so deeply in our unconscious and is protected so well by our ego mind. The woman I described previously with M.S., didn't sit and consciously plan all day long how she was going to use her illness to control her husband. She wasn't even consciously aware she was controlling him with it. She just knew he was now giving her what she had wanted from him for many years. With this state of affairs set up for her by her illness, could I really expect her to want to get well? She has become comfortable being a victim of her illness. It works for her. The freedom her healing promises contains within it the threat of chaos, change, and loss of the dysfunctional arrangement she has been enjoying with her husband. From her perspective, the cost of her healing is more than she is willing to pay.

For me, these patients are the hardest patients to work with because all that is done for them to help them get well is unconsciously sabotaged. They must look like they are working hard to get well because this pacifies their inner conflict but underneath it all, they are frightened of what their healing promises. We don't have to be a patient with an illness to experience this situation. We experience it all of the time with various situations in our lives. We are frightened of who we are and who we can be when we live authentically the fullness of our being. We are frightened of the freedom living so boldly can bring us. Instead we rationalize our victimization and use it to cover up the fact that underneath it all, we are scared to death of our potentialities and possibilities; scared to death of realizing our own power and authority as an individual expression of The Divine.

Creativity Is the True Healer

Chaos appears to be the root of life's creativity as it is described in systems and chaos theory. It functions as a harbinger of change forcing living systems to creatively transform and adapt to that change. When it occurs in our lives, I see chaos as an invitation from life, to change. I have witnessed the illness in people's lives, acting as a chaotic event, inviting them to change their life in some way. The change requested of them is always one requiring them to live more fully; requiring them to live more authentically, more productively, and more compassionately involved with life and the world around them. When we discover the secret fear that holds us back from living more fully, that fear that has kept us trapped in our comfort zone of limited freedom and accountability even when it includes illness, we would do well to face it and overcome it. This demands of us creative thinking.

When we accept life's invitation for greater life and decide to change our lives so we can more fully realize our Light, we must be creative. Creativity gives us the ability to transcend our fear, to transcend traditional ideas, rules, patterns, and relationships that may be limiting and dysfunctional to our growth, keeping us in the cycle of illness. Creativity is "the elixir of life" that heals and transforms life. Through the creative process we enter a sacred place. We enter that zone of evolution where the world lights up to itself as we light up to the world. In the moment we are fully present in the act of creating we are reunited with the magic that gave us birth; reunited with the waters of the wellspring of life. Creativity is the source of the River of Life from which all creative energy and vitality issue forth to be manifested as new life. Through every creative act, life fulfills itself. Therefore, through every creative act we enter into, we transcend the mortality of our three dimensional ego-self and enter the realm of immortality to become one with our greater self; one with The Divine. In the creative act we become a self-realized collaborator with The Divine in the creation of our life story and of the world. Through creativity, we are revitalized and delivered from the chaos of illness into the dynamic order and freedom of a new life.

When I graduated from nursing school in 1976, I began working at The Cleveland Clinic on the post op open heart surgery unit and then infectious diseases intensive care. I worked three different shifts in a week and worked long, stressful hours. I had just broken off a five year engagement with the wedding planned. In my off time, I was being formally trained in western mystical traditions and Jewish Kabbalah. It was a difficult time of much change. I needed the medicine creativity offered me. I needed to paint again! I needed to go back home again where that magic that connected me to something greater than myself existed.

One day, on my way home from work, I bought a large 34" x 52" canvas. I lived in a one bedroom apartment with little space to spare. So I shoved my bed up against the wall and turned it on its side to make room for my painting. I struggled at first, as though I had never painted before, finding myself in a vulgar conversation with an inanimate object . . . my canvas. Then it happened! I broke through the limitations of my limited thinking and began to "feel" the painting on the canvas. The more I felt it, the more it flowed and I painted. I painted all night and into the next morning through my alarm for work. I called in sick and continued painting all day and all night rarely breaking to drink, eat or use the bathroom. I called in sick again and kept painting. I painted for seventy two hours straight without stopping. Better stated, something painted through me for seventy two hours, something of magic.

I accessed something greater than myself when I painted that picture. I stepped outside of who I was in the limited sense of myself caught in my struggle and fear and merged with a greater experience of myself as *Thou*, as The Divine. I became the brush in the hand of a greater artist. I became "the hollow bone," the conduit for the waters of life to flow through. As I painted, I was healed and my life was changed. When we access the magic of creativity we step outside of time and our mortal selves to become immortal for a moment. It doesn't matter what we create; a painting, a garden, a poem, or a bench. Whatever it is we create, it will heal us where we are wounded and free us where we are imprisoned by our fear. Creativity is the true healer. Creativity is our true medicine.

Imagination is essential for creativity. It guides and directs the creative visualization of our healing and wellness. Imagination becomes "the substance of things hoped for" as described biblically in the definition of faith. For us to creatively overcome our fear and change our lives, we will need to employ imagination. It has been said, "What we can imagine, we can accomplish." However, as I have stated earlier, I am astonished at how so many of my patients can't imagine what their life would be like if they were without their illness and fear. Asking them to imagine this is one of the homework exercises I give them and rarely do they accomplish it. It appears to be a difficult task for many of them. The question that comes up here for me is: "Is it that they lack imagination or is it that they unconsciously feel threatened by the possibility of being well?"

The Not So Secret Fear

Paul Tilich tells us, "Fear of death determines the anxiety in every fear." ". . . anxiety in its nakedness, is always the anxiety of nonbeing."[2] I agree with his statement, but find it extremely ironic that the two most primary fears we deal with deep in our psyches are so conflicting. One is the fear of dying and the other is the fear of fully living. We certainly fear dying and becoming nonexistent. There is no doubt about that. This is a fear we openly accept and talk about often: "I have a fear of flying." "I have a fear of drowning." "I have a fear of falling, a fear of cancer, etc." How many times do we here ourselves confess these fears openly? But how often do we hear ourselves say we are afraid of living? "I am afraid to be all that I can be." "I am afraid to be successful." "I am afraid to be healthy or get well."

As I have already shared, I have seen the fear of fully living, regularly play a bigger role in illness more so than the fear of dying. However, both do have a role. When we find ourselves being called by our struggle or our illness to wake up to a change in ourselves that is needed for our continued growth and evolution, we must first find out what fear lies beneath it. To identify the fear that limits us in our struggle and illness is to identify the denizen of our unconscious that needs to be slain; the gift that needs to be sacrificed in the fire of our burning ground. Are we frightened of our death or are we frightened of our power and freedom?

The fear of death will show itself in our resistance to let go of something old and familiar that has served us and is no longer beneficial to our growth. This could be a memory of a wounding, a belief, a relationship, a way of thinking, a lifestyle, or a dietary pattern. Our ego mind will of course protest loudly and try to make a trade for something of less value. Our heart will know what has seen its time. Always, when we let go of something that has served us, we let go of it in gratitude and love for what it has given us. When we slay our dragons they are to be slain with love. When we sacrifice our gifts to the fire of the burning ground they are to be laid upon the fire with gratitude. When we do this in this way, what has served us well will always be a part of us but no longer an obstruction to us.

The fear of our own power and the freedom it brings us will show itself more insidiously. We will make all sorts of excuses as to why we can't do whatever it is we are being called to do for us to live more fully. The tell-tale sign of this fear is what I call the *victim soliloquy*, "I can't because of . . ." "I have no say in this." "It is out of my power." "Such and such made me do it." As I am writing this I am laughing at myself because I'm thinking of how many times I still sing this soliloquy to myself and the world. I am thinking further how much we all must sing this familiar declamation of powerlessness when we are asked to be more and live more who we were born to be in our fullest. I say to you all, when we hear its monotonous oration in our heads and our speech, we should pause a moment and say "the old prayer" to ourselves and then go ahead and change what we can change. As poet Dylan Thomas instructs, "Do not go gentle into that good night. Rage, rage against the dying of the light."[3]

Dr. Patrick Donovan

References

1. Neumann E: *The Origins and History of Consciousness.* Princeton University Press, 1954; 104
2. Tillich P: *The Courage To Be.* Yale Univ. Press, 1952; 38
3. Dylan Thomas: *The Poems of Dylan Thomas.* New Directions Publishing. 1952

Chapter Seven

Celling Our Stories

"Your memory is a monster; you forget—it doesn't. It simply
files things away. It keeps things for you, or hides things
from you—and summons them to your recall with will of
its own. You think you have a memory; but it has you!"
(*John Irving, "A Prayer for Owen Meany"*)

"But who can remember pain, once it's over? All that remains
of it is a shadow, not in the mind even, in the flesh."
(*Margaret Atwood, "The Handmaid's Tale"*)

Outstanding in Our Fields

Our spaces are filled with fields of memory and habitual patterns that link us all with one another and with the world around us, like a spider's webbing. These spatial memory fields are continually influenced by our thoughts, feelings, and the choices we make. In turn, our thoughts, feelings and choices are influenced by these fields. According to numerous studies over the past twenty years, the memory of our life story is likely stored in the memory fields between us and inside of us as well as in our brain. Noted biologist and author Rupert Sheldrake, named these phenomena *morphogenetic fields*.[1] He describes these fields as influencing the form, biological patterning, and cellular structure of all living things. These fields are ancient and yet dynamic because we are all still influencing them and being influenced by them every day. Our stories and the stories of our ancestors appear to be carried in these fields and therefore in our cellular structure as these memory fields influence our cellular patterning and our epigenetic triggering.

We have a cellular memory stored in the cells of our body that doesn't require our brain alone to store it or access it. It is a result if the organizing influence of morphogenetic fields as well as our genetics. Our genes play an essential role in this organizing influence on our cells. However, our genetics are not solely responsible for it or for us being who we are. As a matter of fact, it appears to be the field that influences our genes and their expression and not necessarily the other way around. I theorize Carl Jung's "collective unconscious" may be the evidence of this organizing field of memory at play in our human psyche influencing our actions and reactions to life. The psychological archetypes of this collective unconscious may be the result of age-old patterns or memories in the morphogenetic field of our human consciousness.

From the accumulating evidence of scientific investigation into morphogenetic fields, we are apparently what we choose, what we have chosen, and what our parents and ancestors have chosen. Those choices are written in the morphogenetic field of memory within and around us. Our story is informed and enformed by all of those choices. It is deeply intermingled with the story of others, those of us living in the present and those millions of our ancestors who have long passed from this life. Each one of us is outstanding in our field and the fields of others. As I have indicated earlier, this has its pros and its cons. Its pros are: we are influenced by the memory fields and choices of those around us and those who have come before us. Its cons are: we are influenced by the memory fields and choices of those around us and those who have come before us. We are never alone in the writing of our story. However, we do have the greatest influence on it and its outcomes by how we choose daily to think, feel, and live our life.

The morphogenetic field is sensitive to our intentions and actions. It reacts to our thoughts, actions, and emotional responses like a spider's web reacts to a bug caught in it. As we move through our life unfolding our story, we signal this memory field of our choices and actions and the field responds. It then records this response and restructures the field appropriately in the context of all the other influences affecting it. The structuring and restructuring of this field, in turn influences our continued cellular patterning. Hence, the old saying, "We are what we think." If we continually think depressively, our cells may react depressively; slow to repair and regenerate. If we are always angry, we may experience increased inflammatory reactions in our tissues as well. If we are too fearful of the world around us and over-reactive to it, we may experience environmental sensitivities and allergies to nonthreatening chemicals and natural pollens and molecules. If we continue to live a creatively restrictive life, we may develop cancer as our cells effectively rebel against their restrictions of differentiation to fulfill our unconscious and unrealized wishes for more creative freedom and expression.

I am not saying we are solely responsible for causing our illness and hence should feel guilty for creating it or inferior for having it. What I am saying here, is that the nature of our illness is influenced by the nature of who we are, how we live our lives, and how our ancestors lived. As I have said in Chapter One, we don't get cancer. It arises out of our own cellular makeup. It arises out of who we are. We are our cancer and it is an expression of us, of our cellular dysfunction. I find many people strongly protest this idea. Yet I find few of us having any problem understanding how eating poorly and consuming tons of high-fat foods could cause heart disease. It seems to be OK with most people, considering this example of heart disease, to accept the fact that the outcome of years of bad dietary choices contribute to illness. But it can be considered ridiculous by many of those same people to accept the fact that the outcome of living years with cynical mistrust of other people's motives (such as believing that most people will lie to get ahead), frequent feelings of anger, and aggressive expression of hostility toward others without regard for their feelings makes us much more prone to have a heart attack, for instance.[2] Yet there is evidence for this.

The Issues Are in the Tissues

Accumulating evidence has made it clear that our experience—the knowledge we acquire during a lifetime of sensing and acting—is of fundamental biological relevance to us and our physical body. Our experience makes an impact on all of our adaptive systems, including our endocrine, immune, and nervous systems. It is of the essence, not only for the unfolding of our healthy status, but also for the development of our dysfunctional traits.[3] After decades of research in psychoneuroimmunology, it is finally clear how our emotions create the bridge between our mind and body. What we think and feel is interpreted by our bodies into various molecules (short chains of amino acids called peptides) that become, in our bodies, the biochemical correlates of our emotions.[4] These peptides can be found in our brain as well as our stomach, our muscles, our glands and all our major organ tissues. As we experience assorted emotional responses to various events in our daily lives, those emotions we feel are interpreted into chemical messengers in our bodies, and our bodies respond. Our emotions therefore, affect our physical bodies and visa versa.

Of further interest is the newer science of epigenetics and what it has revealed to us regarding our mind, body, and ancestral connections. We have known for a few decades DNA is the crucible of who we are. It holds the genetic coding for all of our traits and personal characteristics. But what we didn't know until recently is that some genetic regulator outside of the tightly wound spiral of DNA inside each of our cell's nucleus is required to tell our DNA exactly which genes to transcribe and at what times. These genetic regulators are molecules (methyl groups and histones) that are attached to our DNA and not part of its basic internal structure, hence, the term "epigenetics" (outside of our genes). These epigenetic molecules direct and regulate our genetic expression. They control which genes ultimately get expressed. Our cells perform different functions not because they have different DNA, but because they have different patterns of methyl groups and histones controlling which genes in our DNA are expressed at any one time. Thus, although the DNA in each one of our own cells is identical, its epigenetic counterpart is not.[5] It appears to be our epigenomic triggering and influence that affects who we are in our more personally characteristic and novel way of being ourselves.

Our epigenomic influences are different for each individual and family even though our DNA may be nearly identical. Further, our epigenetics are influenced by how we live our lives and how our parents and grandparents lived their lives. That influence is recorded in our epigenome that in turn directs how we express our genetic traits in and through our cellular make up. In other words, our family histories of triumphs and woundings are recorded by our epigenome and passed on to us with our DNA. To paraphrase science writer Dan Hurley, the study of behavioral epigenetics has shown us that traumatic experiences in our past, or in our recent ancestors' past, leave what he calls "molecular scars" adhering to our DNA. He then goes on to say further,

> "Like silt deposited on the cogs of a finely tuned machine after the seawater of a tsunami recedes, our experiences, and those of our forebears, are never gone, even if they have been forgotten. They become a part of us, a molecular residue holding fast to our genetic scaffolding. The DNA remains the same, but psychological and behavioral tendencies are inherited. You might have inherited not just your grandmother's knobby knees, but also her predisposition toward depression caused by the neglect she suffered as a newborn."[6]

The memory patterns of our life story and the stories of our ancestors are written in our morphogenetic memory fields. They are then transcribed onto our genetic and our epigenetic patterning, to finally be expressed into our cellular structure. These memory patterns can be life giving and health promoting or they can be life restricting and illness encouraging. We can choose which it may be for us by how we live our lives; by what fears, woundings, or shadow elements we choose to overcome and sacrifice in the fire of our burning ground and how authentically we choose to dance. Do we hide our light in the darkness of our fear or do we shine it forth to the world? Do we cower in the shadow elements of our woundings or do we live fully becoming all we were born to be? Do we let our illness restrict us or do we let it free us as we use it to guide us into greater healing?

The Idioms of Illness

I have been amazed over the years at how many of my patients will unconsciously choose certain linguistic idioms that describe their illness or its symptoms when explaining a particular life situation. I don't think it is random or inconsequential. I listen carefully for it. To me, this is always a key to the underlying theme of their illness. For instance, I have seen a patient with gastro-esophageal reflux (GERD), also called heartburn, refer to his working situation as something he "could no longer stomach" and thought his boss's rudeness was "too hard to swallow." Hmmm! It's got to make me wonder with this idiomatic, metaphorical association if his work and his boss wasn't the stressor causing his GERD. He didn't have it before working at this job and now he can't stomach it.

Of further interest to me was how, over time, I found this patient himself to be rude. Maybe there was some egoic projection here? Could it be that he was irritated by his own rudeness and his boss was unknowingly acting as his teacher attempting to awaken him to his own shadow element by mirroring this element of rudeness back to him? If so, then is this patient's rudeness a causative factor for his GERD? But then a further question might be, "Why was my patient rude?" What was his ego protecting by his rudeness? What fear or wounding was at play here underneath it all? Whatever it was, I suspect his emotional responses were triggering his reflux and restructuring the cellular response patterning of his memory field to "not stomach what he couldn't swallow;" to not stomach what his ego refused to see. By regurgitating it back up his esophagus, he was physiologically acting out his unwillingness to take it in and digest it.

As I look around at our social and political environment today, I see a lot of us refusing to digest what is happening around us unable to stomach the responsibility of acting on it or doing something about it. At the same time, one of the most common Big Pharma advertisements in the media is for medications to treat our GERD. Is our "refusal to swallow what we can't stomach" or don't want to look at in ourselves now becoming an ingrained memory pattern in our morphogenetic field? Is the human memory field now getting programmed with denial?

When we think of it, much of our language contains idioms. There are estimated to be at least 25,000 idiomatic expressions in the English language alone. An idiom is simply defined as a metaphorical expression whose meaning is not predictable from the usual meaning inferred by its constituent elements or words. Examples of idioms include such phrases as: "He doesn't have the guts." "She's pulling my leg." "They are getting under my skin." "You put your foot in your mouth," It is clear to most of us the actual meaning of the idiomatic phrase is different from the inferred metaphorical meaning or implied meaning. However, in my experience listening to patient's stories, I have witnessed too many times their chosen idiom(s) to ironically match the symptom or illness picture they are coming to see me about, like the man who couldn't stomach his job. Also, when we think of it, how many of our idioms refer to our body parts or functions? Is this because somewhere deep within our morphogenetic field memory or collective unconscious we realize a metaphorical relationship between certain thoughts or emotional issues and specific organs and tissues?

I have come to believe that the metaphorical meanings associated with idioms referencing our body parts or functions are not coincidental. When we "don't have the guts," we are fearful. I have found fear to play an important role in illnesses of the intestinal tract, especially the fear of losing control. Control appears to be a big part of the unconscious energetic underlying inflammatory bowel disease (IBD) and irritable bowel syndrome (IBS). When we "don't have the backbone" or can't "shoulder the weight," we are thought to be too weak and/or too tired to carry our load or our life responsibilities. This weakness and exhaustion from too much responsibility may play a role in the development of osteopenia and osteoporosis. Just think of how an elderly woman with severe osteoporosis walks. She is all hunched over in a way in which any of us would be if we were carrying a heavy load on our back. When a patient "refuses to look at his/her own crap," that patient may end up dealing with chronic diarrhea forced to deal with his/her own crap every day. I can't tell you how many patients with hemorrhoids or musculoskeletal problems have told me something or someone in their life was either a "pain in the butt" or a "pain in the neck." How ironic this all is! I have come to appreciate life's use of irony to make its point clear to us and to facilitate our learning. I have come to know this for myself to be true: Where irony is at work, the Divine Spirit is at play with a mischievous giggle.

SOME COMMON IDIOMS OF ILLNESS

Can't stomach that or don't have the stomach for it
Can't swallow that
Can't shoulder that
Can't see that or I refuse to see that
Pain in the neck, back, ass
Don't have the spine for that
Don't have the guts for that
Thin skinned
Don't have a leg to stand on
Can't handle or grasp that
Give you a piece of my mind

I am speechless
I refuse to hear that
Broken hearted
Inflamed with anger
I have become numb to it
I smell something funny
I have difficulty digesting that
Rash behavior
Full of hot air
Flush with anger/embarrassment
Pulling my hair out over it
No skin off my back
Tight sphinctered or tight assed
Too sensitive/hypersensitive

Killing Our Parents to Free Our Story

Our parents and grandparents have contributed to our story by leaving "molecular scars" on our DNA and memory patterns in our morphogenetic fields, as I discussed earlier. These scars and memories, if unhealthy, can lead us into dysfunctional cellular patterning and illness. Therefore, I suggest we would do well to awaken ourselves to them and work to resolve their negative influences in our lives. This resolution begins with killing our parents. I know this is a strong statement. Of course, I do not mean it literally. I mean it only figuratively or metaphorically. As the fruit drops from the tree and the seed separates from the plant to become its own individual, I have found we are all called upon by life to figuratively kill our parents in the process of growing up healthfully. What I am saying here is we have a responsibility to ourselves and to our family line of origin to accomplish two primary tasks in our lives:

1) To realize the inherited scars and wounding issues of our ancestral line into which we were born and heal them;

2) To free ourselves from our parents' protective and instructional dictates and their subjective influences, prejudices, and beliefs so that we can discover who we are in our authenticity, claim our own personal sovereignty, and then live it fully and creatively.

The second of these two primary tasks is commonly the theme that runs through the teenage years: "It is my life. I will do what I want!" "You don't understand me. Things were different when you were growing up!" "You don't know anything!" "You never let me do anything!" "You are ruining my life!" "I hate you and I hate living in this house!" Do any of these statements sound familiar? Welcome to the teen age monolog of parental murder. It seems to me the better job they do at this as teenagers, the more they realize their independence and the closer they end up being to us as adults and as friends. I remember the day my 14 year old daughter announced I could no longer hug her in public or call her "my peanut." My son boldly announced to me, at the age of thirteen, I couldn't call him my "little man" any longer. All of this was the beginning of my children cutting themselves free of me. Now, my daughter still hugs me without a second thought and calls me daddy when she needs me. She is now twenty eight; a grown woman, my friend and a wise friend at that. My son, well he is seventeen and still pushing hard against me with a strong set of personal ethics and a disdain for incompetent authority, just like someone else I know very well. But he has to discover this for himself with his own style of rebellion. As for my step-son, he is just turning thirteen. We will see. If it were up to me, I would have an ICD-9 code (This is a disease code for billing health insurance companies.) called "teenager." The transient pathology would be understood by all of us immediately and wouldn't need any further explanation.

The story of who we are is intricately interwoven and entangled in the story of our parents both personally and archetypically as we are growing up in our formative years. As we enter our teenage years, our job then becomes one of healthy disentanglement from them. I have found when we don't healthfully disentangle from either of our parents we can carry that parent deeply in our inner space in a negative way. If that parent or our relationship with that parent was unhealthy in any way and was a source of wounding to us through abuse, physical or emotional abandonment, psychiatric dysfunction, and so forth, we will continue that parent's dysfunctional behaviors towards us deep inside ourselves and our subconscious mind. That unhealthy memory or wounding then drives the dysfunctional patterning of our illness and our life. For instance, we will become our own abuser of ourselves if our parent was abusive towards us. We will abandon our dreams, our loved ones, or our responsibilities if we were abandoned.

I had a thirty six year old patient diagnosed with B cell lymphoma who had started his chemotherapy treatments. He came to me to see what I could do to help him through his treatments to reduce side effects and help him reduce his risks for recurrence. He was a lawyer with a bit of an anger issue. I was curious as to where that anger was coming from. As I heard his story and questioned him in greater detail, I found out his first symptom (swollen lymph node in his neck) occurred just after his father's death. He hadn't been talking to his father. His father was "hard on him," used to "take a belt to him in the barn" when he disobeyed his father's dictates or got into trouble. His father was a lawyer and pushed my patient hard to become a lawyer. He was angry at his father for controlling his life yet loved him. He was angry at himself for not talking to his father over many years and now his father was gone. My patient felt guilt, resentment, and anger gnawing away at him inside. Could this have been the energetic source of his cancer? After our first meeting, I told my patient to go back to the farmhouse in Connecticut where he grew up while in the area on a business trip. I wanted him to go back to the barn and have the conversation with his father he never got to have. Apparently, the house had been sold a long time ago when my patient was starting college. I was astonished at his story when he returned. It taught me a lot.

He went to his old house in Connecticut and knocked at the door. The elderly couple who lived there were the original people who bought the house from his parents some eighteen years earlier. The couple actually remembered him. They told him to feel free to explore the old lopsided barn that wasn't ever much used by them. As he entered the old barn his heart was racing. Then he saw it! He saw the actual belt his father used on him. It was still hanging on the same old nail. He dropped to his knees and wept like a child for nearly an hour, holding the belt and talking with his father. He told me later it was the most powerful and healing experience he had ever had in his life. He went on to say, "Something changed in me that day. Something of my father's was put away and finished in me while something else was awakened. I understood how much he really did love me. He loved me the best he knew how and gave me what he thought was the most important lessons for me to be a man. They weren't delivered in the best way. He wasn't taught how to do that very well. None-the-less, it was the best way he knew as his father used to beat him and criticize him without cause. What he gave me was so much better than what his father gave him and what I will give my children will be even better yet."

My patient did well through his chemotherapy and had a good response with full remission. That was sixteen years ago. He has had no further recurrences to my knowledge. Yes. The chemotherapy and the nutritional and dietary treatments helped him through his physical illness but so did his experience in the old barn. He now could go on living knowing he was truly loved by his father. He healed and resolved a long-standing familial paternal pattern of abuse, anger, and resentment. He placed his father's belt on the fire of his burning ground and with it, his anger and resentment. He placed the belt with love and walked away from the dance changed. He was healed. So many of us have old barns, belts, nails, and more we haven't yet placed on our fires. Some of us reluctantly hold on to them because in some dysfunctional way they give us comfort and security and often provide the excuse we need to not risk our life for greater life. They can keep us ill. They can be the slow death of us if we are not careful.

What Have Our Fathers Kept for Us?

In 2007, I found myself caught in between as both a father and a son. I was caught in the purgatory of attempting to heal my father's wounds and its lineage of pain while doing my best not to pass them down to my then fourteen year old son who was facing his own struggles. My father was dying slowly in an Alzheimer's care facility. He no longer knew me, his only child. After a few years of sever dementia and my mother's death, he became acutely ill with pneumonia and was dying in a hospital room. I was with him nearly 24/7 for those last few days, watching him struggle to stay alive. He was a fighter all his life and a proud man who would never have wanted this for himself or the ones he loved. I was confused and couldn't understand why he kept holding on to life for so long in this state of dementia and with mom gone. Then something of magic happened. He became present and aware for a moment and called out my name as if searching for me after a couple years of not remembering me at all. "Pat, Pat!" I spoke into his ear, "I am here dad." His whole body relaxed for a moment. He knew me. He was home again for a moment. I then spoke softly, "Dad, mom is gone. She is waiting for you on the other side. I am fine here. I'll be OK dad. I want you to go be with mom again." (My parents were a "unit" for sixty three years.) Then what he said to me healed me and transformed me. It healed the field memory of my lineage and my life. He said clearly with such concern, "I can't leave you Pat!" At that moment I finally understood why he held on for so long even in the state he had been in. The old soldier he was couldn't abandon his last and most important charge. He couldn't leave me. He couldn't leave his only child; his only son. He passed away a few hours later alone, during one of the only few times I left his bedside.

WHAT HAVE OUR FATHERS KEPT FOR US?

What have our fathers kept for us in some secret place we have not yet discovered?

I know of "things" kept in such secret places.

As a son:

I know of disheveled sock drawers that smell of my father, full of old letters, faded baby pictures, crayon-colored father's day cards, broken watches, rusted pocket knives, and elementary school report cards . . . sacred souvenirs of a life's story . . . moments of contemplative remembrances that sweeten a father's soul and confirm the value of his work.

I know of moldy boxes on forgotten shelves of a garage full of old metal toys and tattered-cornered children's books . . . the sources of many night time stories of secret treasures and hidden places in themselves, stories told between the lucid moments of a father's hard worked day and the snores from sleep's incessant demands on his time.

I know of closets full of old "shiny" suits, worn shoes and cuffed pants that jingle with the sound of pocketed change . . . the remnants of forgotten possibilities . . . priceless handouts often used to win a little boy's heart so excited to see his father home.

I know of a courageous man's secret heart places where a little boy still misses his mother who died and left him alone when he was nine . . . where a grown man still weeps like that child when he remembers the horror of war and "his buddies" who died beside him. He cries, "Why not me?" He still holds the guilt. It has aged him.

I know the darkest of secret places where an aged, brittle body with a demented brain holds the soul of a loving man captive in the terrifying darkness of aloneness and the lovelessness of a memoryless, Alzheimered existence. There is no little boy here any longer . . . no drawers . . . no boxes . . . no closets. There are no stories here anymore.

As a father:

I know of disheveled sock drawers that smell of my son full of old Pokemon cards, pencil erasers, half-eaten hard candies, and stones from an adventure on the beach with dad.

I know of disorganized closets full of game boards and boxes, bats and balls, favorite sweat shirts that no longer fit, and shoes of all kinds for all manner of events all thrown together as if in a blender to be mixed into a smoothie of a little boy's delights.

I know of testosterone places no longer secret and hidden where little boys are sacrificed on alters of time and men are erected into platinum statues of arrogant gods who have all of the answers but none of the right questions and none of the grit.

And I know of the darkest of secret places where a son's heart grieves the slow, indignant death of a father and a father's soul aches at the emptiness of his son's room. No little boy here any longer, no father as well; no drawers, boxes, closets or bedtime stories anymore.

P. Donovan, 2009

A GUY PLACE

It is interesting, the alchemy a son experiences at the death of his father. The quick-silver of a little boy is instantly transmuted into the precious gold of a grown man no matter what age he might be at his father's passing. Fathers hold a special place for sons as they do for daughters. But the place for sons is different. It's a "guy place." It's a place filled with integrity, courage and honor; 30 second anecdotes for living and endless "rules of the road"; bedtime stories of heroes and dragons and little boy things . . . timeless remembrances of a father's love for a son such as pocket knives and baseball cards, old stamps and elementary school report cards, cigar boxes of high school letters and a father's day card from an eighth grade hell-dell. When a father dies, the little boy things he held so dearly for his son also die leaving only a man standing alone on his own . . . a man with 30 second anecdotes of life, stories of heroes, and integrity and courage all of his own.

P. Donovan, 2010

When we "kill our parents" we must do it with love. When we do, we will discover the gifts of love they have given us even if those gifts are few. Then, that love heals us. It sets us free to discover who we are unencumbered by the scars and woundings. If we kill our parents with anger and resentment, we will breed greater illness within us and between us and the ones we love. If we do not kill our parents at all, we may die a slow death of dysfunctional entanglement never fully realizing ourselves. Sometimes I have wondered if the actual killings of parents that have made the news, done by angry and confused teens, were not the outer expression of this metaphorical act when the true psychological outlet wasn't accessible to them for whatever reasons.

Fruit can rot on the tree never producing a new tree with fruit of its own. The fruit and its seed must be fully freed from the tree so that it can journey out and populate an orchard or a forest. I have seen so much healing begin with this first step of identifying the familial scars and woundings that hold us back from fully self-realizing and living our individual story to its fullest. There are things from our families and our parents worth keeping and valuing. We don't need to go looking for them. They will show themselves clearly to us when we live our lives fully. There are things from our families and parents we should not keep. They are to be place in the fire of our burning ground with love so we can let them turn into ashes and smoke.

References

1. Sheldrake R: *A New Science of Life: The Hypothesis of Formative Causation.* J.P. Tarcher, 1981
2. Raymond C: "Distrust, rage may be 'toxic core' that puts 'type A' person at risk." *JAMA*, 1989: 261; 813
3. Ulvestad E: "Psychoneuroimmunology: the experiential dimension." *Methods Mol Biol.* 2012; 934: 21-37
4. Pert C: *Molecules Of Emotion.* Simon & Schuster, N.Y., 1992
5. Hurley D: "Grandma's Experiences Leave a Mark on Your Genes." *Discover.* May, 2013
6. Ibid.

Chapter Eight

Fiction or Nonfiction

"People don't want to hear the truth because
they don't want their illusions destroyed."
(*Friedrich Nietzsche*)

"Remembrance of things past is not necessarily
the remembrance of things as they were."
(*Marcel Proust*)

"To see the Real for what it is requires being able to discern
error, which is the unintentional mistaking of the Real, as well
as deception, which is the intentional use of error or imposition
of error. Error imposed by intention becomes the Lie."
(*John Lamb Lash, "Not In His Image"*)

Fictional Stories

Often what we remember emotionally from an event
in our life that has caused us wounding isn't the true
story. It is commonly a mixture of a truth and a false
conclusion; one-half is true regarding the details of the actual
event and one-half is fiction regarding our interpretation of and
emotional response to the actual event. Consider for instance,
my patient who suffered with chronic depression, fibromyalgia
(FM), and performance anxiety. She was haunted with the
feelings of inadequacy causing her to feel as though she wasn't
worthy of being loved. Her associated physiological illness was

FM with which she was formally diagnosed. There was clearly a nondescript autoimmune inflammatory component to her FM as demonstrated in her blood work. When we discussed various stressors in her life she used the idiom of, "I'll just have to iron all that out." After putting this together, what did I have?

I had a patient who was inflamed at herself (autoimmunity) and attacking herself in a way that caused her generalized pain in her muscles and joints. This pain inhibited her from doing a lot of things; the work at home she needed to do as well as her job. This was interesting to me because she reported having performance anxiety; anxiety about doing anything due to the fear she was going to "mess up" and "do it all wrong." This pain from her FM, then subconsciously gave her reason to not do the work she needed to do. It also gave her an excuse as to why she did "mess up" if she did the work poorly. The pain of FM, in its dysfunctional way, was working for her as was her illness. Her depression caused her to isolate herself further assuring no one would see her mess up. Her subconscious fear of living, of risking life for greater life, was more than her fear of isolation and death. She had chosen isolation and a slow death over life. As I questioned her much more thoroughly to explore the causative wounding(s) that may have led her into this dysfunctional predicament, a very interesting story emerged.

Apparently, at about the age of six, she was helping her mother iron clothes. Her mother left her for a moment to go to the bathroom. Excited and happy to be helping her mother, she took her mother's favorite blouse out of the pile of freshly washed clothes and put it on the ironing board. She was going to show her mommy what a good job she could do. She ironed the blouse holding the iron down on it for too long of a time. Needless to say, she ruined the blouse. When her mother returned and saw the results of this little girl's attempt to do something special for her mommy, she screamed at her daughter repeatedly, "You just can't do anything right, can you? I leave you alone for just a few moments and what do you do? You ruin my best blouse. I just can't trust you to do anything right." For a little girl whose mother is everything primary in her life at that time, this was a devastating wounding. She has spent her life trying to "iron it out."

Now what is the truth and what is the fiction of this story? The truth is this: she ruined her mother's best blouse trying to do something nice for her mother. The fictional aspect of this story is: she can't do anything right especially for the people she loves and if she tries and fails, they will emotionally abandon or scold and criticize her. Loving her wasn't worth anybody's time because she will just end up failing them. This fictional story arose because a six year old girl can't rationalize out the facts. "I did my best to help my mommy and just made a simple mistake because I didn't know the proper way to iron a blouse. No one had taught me how yet. Mommy just got angry for a minute but still loves me anyway. I'll just learn how to iron properly and do a better job next time. We all make mistakes as we learn."

My patient's false story, based on her "wounded" interpretation of the event, got attached to her true story. It was then imprinted in her morphogenetic field memory and cellular patterning to later emerge as FM, depression, and autoimmunity. She hadn't successfully identified this source wounding in her life and certainly hadn't successfully killed her mother. Instead, she actually took over for her mother as many of us do. She took over her mother's sharp criticism and turned it onto herself as autoimmunity. She was angry at herself for what she did and continued to blame herself. This was the primary wounding energetic that fueled her illness and it wasn't true at all. It was a fictional story that became a groove in an unconscious broken record playing over and over in every life situation she encountered.

How many broken records play in all of our stories? What is the repeating idiom or reiterated monolog of struggle each one of us spews on a daily basis? Answering this question can lead us to a false story of wounding that may be feeding our dysfunction and illness. Remember, that false story can be our false story or it can be an echo pattern of our parents' and grandparents' fictional story held in our morphogenetic field and epigenetic memory.

Unintentional Error and Illusion

According to very ancient teachings from the Gnostic oral traditions and writings (Nag Hammadi Library) as well as Sanskrit and Buddhist concepts of illusion, our capacity to error is intrinsic to being human and to the process by which we learn and evolve. Our error occurs in our interpretation of our experiences and perceptions of the world around us. This error in our interpretation then leads to illusion. Our illusion then creates a false story and that false story fills our spaces and conditions our memory fields and epigenetics. Our illusion is not a result of our perception of the world or ourselves. It is instead a result of our "false interpretation" of our perception. The Buddhist scholar H. V. Guenther clarifies this: "Illusion does not mean the illusion of perception, but the false conclusion we base on perception."[1] How we interpret our experiences and perceptions of the world and at what conclusions we arrive (either false or true), is based on two primary conditions: 1) our ability to "know ourselves" and clearly discern our unintentional mistaking of the "Real" and then correct it and; 2) our ability to clearly discern when our unintentional mistaking of the Real has been intentionally imposed upon us as deceit so we can then call it out in its truth.

Discernment is the key that allows us to do this. It is the tool that frees us from our error of illusion.

To discern is to detect with our senses something as separate or distinct from something else and come to realize and understand the differences. For us to discern the real from the false in our stories, the nonfictional from the fictional, we are required by the definition of discernment to recognize and understand the differences between them. A simple but good example of this might be if we were waiting for a new date to pick us up at our home. Our date was to be there at seven o'clock and it is now seven thirty. He hasn't contacted us at all and we are concerned he forgot or just isn't coming. We begin to make up stories based on our woundings: "I knew he wouldn't show up. How could he be interested in me? I am a fool for thinking this could work." Another scenario might be this: "He looked like one of those smooth talkers. He was just leading me on. He is so irresponsible to not call me, etc." Then the doorbell rings. It is your date. He is standing at the door with a policeman and he is a mess. He was mugged on the way to your house and his phone and car were stolen. The officer states, "Mam, he wanted me to take him here because he was concerned about you waiting." Now how would we feel . . . a bit embarrassed? Simple discernment at this moment would quickly show us our false stories and we would have a choice. We could accept the truth and let go of our fictional stories made up from our false conclusions of a real event or we could hold on to them and tell our date to just leave and not come back again.

This is a simple example of how we would apply discernment when faced with the error of our false interpretation. In reality, however, it isn't quite this simple. It is usually much more complex and confusing. Discerning the Real from our false conclusions IS one of the hardest tasks life requires of us. This discernment is

NOT easy by any account. Just when we think we have gotten it right, we discover otherwise. However, according to so many great minds through the ages, mystics, theologians, and philosophers alike, this task of discernment is thought to be one of our primary tasks in life. I have to agree with this. I have certainly witnessed our lack of this discernment, our error in interpreting our experiences and perceptions, to be the primary source of illness.

Consider further my patient with FM who errored in her interpretation of the ironing event with her mother. She was six years old. Can we really expect a six year old little girl to discern correctly at the complex level required to realize what was real and what was "made up" by her emotional interpretation of her scolding event? Of course we can't. Therein lies her wounding. This is why so many of our major woundings occur in childhood and hold such a deep, lasting, subconscious grip on us. They stay with us a long time and become so ingrained in our subconscious we cannot easily see them consciously and are not aware of them. However, they drive our behavior and responses in every relationship and emotional event in our life until we are able to see them and change them.

As we emotionally experience traumatic events later in our lives as adults, we would think we would be more capable of applying discernment and realizing what is true about the traumatic event and what is errored interpretation on our part. However, by this time, our ego mind is well developed and will employ any and all means it can to keep us free from fear, risk, and vulnerability. Therefore, the nonfictional stories it will make up to keep us safe from that fear, risk and vulnerability, may still be hard to discern. Remember, our ego is a trickster and will use our own discernment tools to trick us into believing our own nonfictional story as true and rationalize to no end why that is so. How many of our "stories" about ourselves, our parents and children, our friends and lovers, and the world we live in are fictional, based on our unintentional error of false conclusions? How many of these same stories have led us into the mire of unintended consequences resulting in pain, heartache, and illness?

Our lives are filled with the risk of error. However, the "error" I am referring to here is not the error associated with the ego judgment of right or wrong. It is the error referred to in Buddhist and Gnostic teachings as the "error of false conclusions that leads to unintended consequences." In these teachings, there is no right or wrong. There is simply choice and the consequences and outcomes as a result of that choice offering opportunity for further choices. The consequential "further choices" then present us with a chance to correct our error. Correcting our error simply means making new choices that give us consequences with which we are happy and content and offer us the possibility of greater growth and evolution. Think about it though. If we do not risk error, we may not live fully to appreciate life in its fullness.

There is a story of a student monk in a Buddhist monastery who was struggling with a situation. Every morning the senior monk would see his student in the garden emotionally wrestling with himself and pacing the garden for hours. Finally, the elder monk approached his student in the garden and asked, "Student, why do you struggle so?" The student replied, "Master, I am faced with a situation and need to make a choice as to how to proceed and don't want to make the wrong decision. I want to make the right decision." The master then replies, "Student, why do you struggle so?" The student again says, "I am faced with a situation and need to make a choice as to how to proceed and don't want to make the wrong decision. I want to make the right decision." Again the master asks, "Student, why do you struggle so?" Well, the student is now fully confused and frustrated. He is wondering why the elder monk isn't hearing his answer and so he asks the senior monk, "Why is it you are not hearing my answer to your question? I keep telling you why I am struggling!" The master then replies, "Student, why is it you continue to struggle with the right or wrong choice? There is no "right" or "wrong." There simply is a choice and the resultant consequences of that choice. If you do not like the consequences, simply make another choice." There is no error, only opportunity. When we are accountable to ourselves, our error is always filled with opportunity for new directions because it offers us new choices.

Intentional Error and Deceit

Our ancestors constructed mythological stories in an attempt to explain the primary cause of error leading to dysfunction and illness in the human condition. According to ancient Gnostic teachings and Western Abrahamic traditions, there is another source of error. It is a primary source that plays a role in creating our false stories. This is deceit; the "intentional" error imposed upon us through a lie. We see this idea theologically introduced and played out in the Western Abrahamic traditions (Judeo-Christian-Islamic) with the mythological story of the devil in the Garden of Eden. In this well-known story, the devil deceives Eve into eating the apple from the Tree of Knowledge of Good and Evil. This is considered the "fall of man" and the first or original sin. According to this metaphorical tale of The Fall of humanity, we were first created pure and innocent and then we participated in an intentionally-imposed false story that appealed to our ego mind, a story of immortality, god-like knowledge and power. When Adam and Eve took a bite of the apple, they succumbed to deceit. Deceit then, by the mythological meaning of this story, is the primary place where we go wrong by falling under the power of deceit, self-imposed and otherwise.

In the ancient Gnostic teachings, the older root of Western thought, we are told a similar story of deceit and error but from a more cosmological conceptualization. According to these teachings, when the Great Mother source of this galactic creation, the Aeon Sophia, plunged unilaterally from the galactic core and poured her massive, self-aware currents of immense pulsations of light and self-ordering consciousness into the unorganized and chaotic realm of darkness, an anomaly or "error" occurred.[2] This error was due to her over-exuberance caused by her ecstatic joy of creating. Because of her over-exuberance, she prematurely plunged herself into the chaos of matter impacting the dense elementary field arrays of the galactic limbs not following the "usual" order of cosmic process. This was the original "unintentional" error that programmed our struggle in this existence.

This error of the great Sophia mother, caused a premature animation of the very dense matter to arise as an inorganic life-form absent of its own innate creativity and originality. It is taught that this inorganic life form was a cosmic aberration as it did not arise from the Sophia's divine substance of pure Organic Light from the central sun. This aberrant life form is referred to in the Gnostic literature as Archons. Archons are described as an alien force that intrudes subliminally upon the human mind, like the devil in Abrahamic mythology, to deviate our intelligence away from its proper and sane applications. Archons attach themselves to our emotional structure and intentionally deviate our thinking into believing false stories. In a sense, they introduce, become, and maintain our false stories and are thought to be the source of our religious and sociocultural false stories that keep us imprisoned in restrictive, uncreative, and conformist thinking for the sake of control.

I find these two stories relevant because they mythologically convey to us what I think is a psychological truth about our human condition that commonly leads to illness. They inform us that deceit is an abnormal condition of our psyche, of our human consciousness and that this abnormal condition creates dysfunction and illness when we succumb to it. As a matter of fact, what we learn from these mythologies is that deceit IS the "primary cause" of dysfunction and illness in our lives. Further, they also convey to us the idea that deceit arises out of our egoic realm of consciousness. Therefore, the greatest deceit we deal with is our own self-deceit. This is the result of our "intentional" constructing of false stories and/or our "unquestioning acceptance" of them to keep us from facing and overcoming the fear of our own light; our fear of living fully and authentically. Denial, for instance, is a great source of such false stories. It does a great job keeping us from being accountable and fully living in our authenticity. Living authentically means living without the self-deceit of "intentional" error. It does not, however, mean living without "unintentional" error. Our capacity to unintentionally error is intrinsic to being human and to the process of our growth. What we also learn from these mythic stories is that intentionally deceiving ourselves and others is not intrinsic to being human or to living healthfully. It is also certainly not intrinsic to loving.

I am the first to admit, it isn't easy to go through life without deceiving our self in some way about something or being deceived into believing the false stories of the many religious, cultural, and socio-political dogmas that exist in our world. Sometimes we just have to push ourselves to purge ourselves of our illusions, both those intentionally and unintentionally imposed upon us. How many of us are "born into" a religion and just buy into its doctrines without even questioning for a moment what our personal truths are and if our truths match with the fundamental teachings of that religion? All of us are, of course, born into a specific sociocultural construct. How many of us just go through life accepting it as our own without exploration or questioning? Many of these religious and sociocultural constructs were created by a person or group of people in a time not relevant to now out of an emotionally traumatic event. Who is to say the resulting story isn't a half-truth constructed from a false conclusion leading to an illusion? Then there is the thought that many of these same constructs were intentionally created to control us and keep us from realizing our full potential and freedom as a co-creator with The Divine.

I find illness to commonly be the evidence of our struggle to purge ourselves of our false stories that restrict our lives or cause us to live in self-deceit and illusion. As I have said earlier in this book, every healing requires a death of some kind. That death then acts as a kind of "rebooting" back to the truth of our primary programming. Just like our computer, when we get locked in a program that isn't working, the first thing we do is to reboot. The reboot is like a death. It resets our computer and allows us to restart anew. If after the reboot, our program continues to malfunction, leading to undesirable consequences, we remove the program and replace it with a new program that is in concert with the truth of our computer and our desired outcome. Like dysfunctional programs, our false stories commonly need to be removed so our healing can be realized. Our figurative rebooting then requires us to deconstruct our stories, look for the dysfunctional errors hidden in them (intentional and unintentional), remove the self-deceit and illusion, and then reconstruct our stories anew into our authentic life story of healing and full self-realization.

Fictional Stories and Characters of Truth

I would like to say a word here about myth. Our human psyche loves stories. It loves making them, telling them and listening to them. Stories are a large part of our history and culture and the most profound of these stories are those of myth. Myths are fictional stories of truth. They are stories that are generally fictional in content and character but factual in theme. Myth is a language all its own. It is a sensual, experiential, and archetypal language of the collective unconscious. Its images and archetypes are universal symbols that speak to our collective unconscious or ancestral morphogenetic memory field. This is where the consciousness and memory of the collective human soul resides. The language of myth is experienced deep in our spaces of awareness. Its images and archetypes stimulate deep internal memories as they stir emotion and feeling. More so, myth is timeless. It lives in the past, present and future but is always experienced in the present moment as its images and archetypes represent ancient truths and primary patterns that are eternally relevant and always applicable to our living.

In mythical stories, it isn't important if the characters were real or not or if the story is based on some sort of historical fact. What matters is the theme of the story. For instance, in the many resurrection myths from Osiris to Jesus Christ, what matters most is the resurrection not who was resurrected or where or when. When we make the "who" important, we miss the point and give our power away in worshipping a hero, a thing. The theme of resurrection, of life passing through death into greater life is what is true and important. This is the principle of continuous creation as I have discussed earlier in the book. It doesn't matter if it is a tree that dies in the forest providing its body for the emergence and growth of new seedlings or if it is the emergence of a caterpillar from its chrysalis, now a butterfly. The mythological story acts as a vehicle for communicating the fundamental life process hidden within its narrative. We can exchange characters and locations but the fundamental theme remains true. Then when we plug ourselves into the story, into the process, WE become the hero/heroine and we then participate in it.

Finally, mythic stories are permissive stories as opposed to restrictive stories. Myths leave infinite room for personal interpretation and participation. Mythic stories encourage our own individual and personal experiences of them. As we hear them told, we realize we are living their mythic theme in our own life. Hence, we become the character in the mythic story because the character in the mythic story already lives in our story as a part of us. Every mythic story and image encourages our active participation in its Divine mystery as it speaks to us through the intuitive, integrative, instinctive, and emotional parts of ourselves that are linked to The Divine. Myth is not fiction. It is the truth of life processes cloaked in the fictional literary fabric of characters and places. As the mythologist Joseph Campbell reminds us, "Wherever the poetry of myth is interpreted as biography, history, or science, it is killed."

Archetypes are another important aspect of myth. All the characters in mythic stories are metaphorical representations of some aspect of our own psyche, of our collective unconscious. They may not have been "real" characters in the sense that they were real people who did everything attributed to them. They are characterizations of original patterns of natural processes and psychological functions that are imprinted within our collective human morphogenetic field. They are thought to be derived from the experiential memories of our race and species. Swiss psychiatrist Carl Jung believed that archetypes are models of people, behaviors or personalities. He believed these models are innate, universal and hereditary and act to organize how we interpret our experiences and perceptions of life. They influence our internal story-making because they are a part of us contributing to the story.

As with all myth, the personage of the archetype is unimportant. What is important is the archetype and how it behaves. For instance, the fact that I am Patrick Donovan is far less important than the fact that I am father. The Archetype of "father" is universal and needs little explanation or definition. On the other hand, the person of "Patrick" is not universal in meaning and understanding and does need definition and clarification. Few people know me and can relate to me. I am not universal, but Father is universal. Father exists in the collective unconscious of our human psyche and experience. I do not. When we "kill our parents" as I discussed in chapter seven, we are really disentangling the person from the archetype; disentangling Patrick from father or Mary from mother. It then makes it easier for us to understand Patrick and Mary for who they are in the "realness" of their stories and in their light and shadow. It helps us to appreciate and love them in a more organic and real sense. When we are done disentangling them from father or mother they are set free. Then, "Set free they step forth in their singleness and confront us as Thou," and we can love them as Patrick or Mary. Their stories are written in our epigenetics and morphogenetic fields while their archetypes live in our collective unconsciousness. We learn much from them.

References

1. Guenther, HV: *Yuganaddha* (Varanasi: Chowkhumba Sanskrit Series, 1969), 64
2. Lash, JL: *Not In His Image.* Chelsea Green Publishing, Vermont, 2006

Chapter Nine

The Hero You
Mythed Was You

"If you are not the hero of your own story, then you're
missing the whole point of your humanity."
(*Steve Maraboli, "Unapologetically You: Reflections
on Life and the Human Experience"*)

"You didn't get the quest you wanted,
you got the one you could do."
(*Lev Grossman, "The Magician King"*)

"Heroes are made by the paths they choose,
not the powers they are graced with."
(*Brodi Ashton, "Everneath"*)

The Hero with Your Face

Our story of healing is a story of self-discovery and
self-affirmation. When we live it fully, our story then
becomes the hero's story as it is told in the mythic stories
of so many cultures and peoples around the world. Discovering
ourselves and our purpose through our illness journey becomes
the transformational element of this story that heals us as we
heal the world. The hero myth best represents our healing
process because its common theme is one of healing. It is one of
resurrection into greater life through the death that transforms

life. It gives us instruction on how best to accomplish this healing resurrection. The hero myth informs us that our healing requires a death of some kind so that we may resurrect into new life. It also informs us that there is no one hero or heroine. We are all the heroes and heroines of our own life stories if we choose to live this transformational hero journey.

As I said in chapter eight, the truth of the hero myth isn't discovered in the character of the hero or the place or time of the story. The truth of this myth is revealed to us through the process the hero must undergo to become the hero. This is the process of death and resurrection that allows for life's continuous creation and evolution. This process is what is important to us to know. It is the true message of the myth. It is exemplified in the mythic story to teach us this fact. Our instruction in this process is made clear to us through the symbolism of the story and its characters. The whole purpose of the hero myth is to convey this truth of healing to us and to be our guide. It isn't to teach us about a historical character, time or place.

The personage of the hero is not important and is replaceable by any one of us as is the time and place of the story. When we focus on the hero and make the hero important as the center piece and message of the myth, we then make a major mistake. We begin to factualise the story itself as true and then worship the hero of that story. This externalizes our own power as we invest it in a personage outside of ourselves and then end up following that person instead of discovering our own unique path of destiny and inspiring others by living it. When this externalization of our power occurs through hero worship, the whole purpose and power of the myth is then lost. The hero myth is designed to apply to all of us at any time or place because it is a universal story of heroic struggle and transformation all of us experience on some level. It invites us all to participate in its universal story and is meant to empower each one of us as we follow its lead and become the hero in our own life story. When we view the mythic story this way, it remains ageless and forever applicable providing us with direction and explicit insight into our collective human psyche . . . our collective human soul and the fundamental processes of nature that influence its function and our healing.

Since each one of us partakes in the process of continuous creation daily in some way, each one of us then becomes the hero in our own story as we live its mythic truth in our lives. Herein lays the beauty of myth. Its story applies to all of us. Each one of us is the pre-hero or the "commoner" born of a miraculous birth (all birth is miraculous) who must undertake a perilous journey (life itself) replete with some great deed of self-sacrifice through which our life is healed and we are transformed into The Hero. When we are ill, our illness provides us with this requisite "perilous journey." The discovery and "slaying" of our shadow elements that obstruct us from living fully; the surrendering of our old and self-restricting stories to the fire of our burning ground and; the conversion of our fictional stories of illness into authentic, self-affirming life stories of healing and transformation serves us as our great deed. Through this great deed we are made whole again. Through this great deed we become the hero or heroine of our own story and live the truth of myth. We then make myth real.

According to psychologist, Erich Neumann, "The transformation of the hero through the dragon fight is a transfiguration, a glorification, indeed an apotheosis, the central feature of which is the birth of a higher mode of personality."[1] As so many of my patients repeatedly have reported to me over the years, the illness they struggled through as their "dragon fight" was the best thing that ever happened to them. It bore for them "a higher mode of personality" by allowing them new self-revelational insights, personal growth, and positive life changes. It became their healing story, their own mythic story of transformation and resurrection. It is now their life story and they are the heroes and heroines of that story because they are healed. All we have to do to make this hero story "our story" of healing is, as Joseph Campbell instructs us, ". . . follow the thread of the hero-path. And where we had thought to find an abomination, we shall find a god; where we had thought to slay another, we shall slay ourselves; where we had thought to travel outward, we shall come to the center of our own existence; where we had thought to be alone, we shall be with all the world."[2]

The Thread of the Hero Path

What is the thread of the hero path? The thread of the hero path is the mythic instruction for personal transformation and healing found in the hero story. As we explore this question, the thread becomes clear as the essential characteristic of the hero/heroine archetype emerges. In all mythic stories the hero gives his life to something greater than himself. Following this mythic instruction then, so should we. Giving of our lives to something greater than ourselves must become an essential characteristic we are to employ for our story of healing to be realized. However, as the hero myth goes on to instruct us, in the giving of our lives to something greater, we may lose our life in some way. A sacrifice is required of us as if to pay the price for our healing. But what is sacrificed? As the myth goes on to instruct us, our life is sacrificed as it is lived inauthentically with all of its illusions and fictional stories of limitation.

As we follow the thread of our mythic story further, we also find out the hero must leave the safety and comfort of home to begin his journey of self-sacrifice and transformation. This is precisely because he must break new ground for himself and for the overall human journey of evolving consciousness and awareness. We learn from this that our old ways of living and thinking that no longer serve our continued growth and evolution must be surrendered to the fire of our burning ground so that out of their ashes new understandings and realizations may arise in us. The hero's journey away from home is a quest founded in love and service. It is not a quest of greed for some self-serving reward. It is marked by a quest for something of great worth that has been lost or for something valuable for the protection or healing of the hero's people, family or culture. It is something elemental and magical with the power to transform and heal. The quest for this magical element always involves difficult trials, struggles, and perilous adventures. When we are at our wit's end with struggles and trials, we would do well to take comfort in knowing we are well into the full throws of our own mythic adventure in which something magical is about to appear to us.

The hero is always tested, often by confrontations with monsters and dragons he must slay. They are manifestations of his own shadow elements and symbolic of ours. His heart and his truth are also tested as he engages various distractions that threaten to take him off course from his goal. As the myth applies to us, these distractions are representative of our own ego mind as it attempts to convince us with all sorts of intellectual rationalizations and reasons why we should not proceed on our quest. It tries hard to keep us safe from the risk of death and the magic of realizing our *Thou* self while keeping us secure in our old ways of being ill. I have seen so many of my patients distracted like this, distracted by their own rationalizations as to why they really don't need to change their diet, exercise more, get their surgery, or take their medicine, or whatever it might be. We live with so many distractions, so many excuses, and so little magic in our lives because of it.

In most hero myths, the hero dies and in his death, he descends to the place of death itself. In his dark gestation there he is faced with terrors and demons. This is symbolic of our own descent into the darkest reaches of our subconscious where we confront the terrors and demons of our woundings and their resultant illusions and false stories. They are to be overcome by us and our fictional stories are to be changed into new stories of truth like the hero who must tame his demons or eliminate them. While buried in this fertile soil of his inner being and facing down his demons, the hero is gestated into new life and arises reborn anew. He emerges healed carrying with him or within him the magic element he was questing after for the healing of his people and his land. For us in this dark place and the dark times of our struggles, we are to realize and manifest our light. We are to see the truth of our stories and reclaim them as ours so that we may arise reborn anew into the light of our truth and then carry that light with us into the world.

Following the lead of the hero story further, at some point through the journey of our personal illness, we are confronted with death. We are asked to undergo some form of therapy that simulates a dying process or a loss. It could be chemotherapy, surgery, or a major change in our life style and diet. Surgery certainly imitates this dying process the most. When we undergo surgery, we are put into a deep anesthetic sleep simulating death while some part of us is removed, is cut out. Then we awake different. With chemotherapy, we are given a known poison to kill our cancer cells and destroy our tumor that is really an aspect of our self. Many of my patients have said going through chemotherapy was like dying. When it comes to drastically changing our lifestyle or diet, we must say goodbye to an old way of living or eating and the mindset and comfort that goes with it. Each one of these situations is a type of death. Like the hero, we often face the demons of our own false stories and fears as we pass through these various therapeutic deaths. Also like the hero, we emerge from these experiences changed, different, and healed carrying the magic element of our healing within in us. But, there is a final question begged by our healing story at this point. It speaks to the cost of our healing. That question is best revealed and understood by the Arthurian hero myth of King Arthur.

Who Does the Grail Serve?

In the Arthurian hero myth of King Arthur, Percival is the Knight of the Round Table who finds the Holy Grail. He is androgynous in his presentation, symbolic of any of us, male or female, who undertake a life-changing, healing quest. As with myth, we are all meant to picture ourselves as Percival no matter our gender. In short, Percival had a vision that the Holy Grail could heal Camelot and so he began his quest along with the rest of the Round Table knights, to realize his vision and find the Grail. It was a quest of love, not of self-gratification. Camelot had become a desolate wasteland with its king wounded and the hearts of its people in darkness. It needed to be healed and by his vision of the Grail, Percival knew the grail could heal it. On his quest for the Grail, Percival finds the Castle of the Holy Grail after much struggle and personal error. In the Castle he is confronted with a question. He sees the wounded King and the glowing cup and because of his compassion for the King and concern for the King's wounding, he is asked, "Who does the Grail serve?" Percival answers, "The Grail serves the people and the land." This was the correct answer. The kingdom was then restored and the king was healed.

Using this mythic hero story as our guide here, I will ask the question in a more relative form regarding our own healing: "Who does our healing serve?" According to Percival's answer, "Our healing is to serve the people and the land." In other words, "Our healing is to serve life." Serving life then becomes our payment for our healing. Once we are healed and begin to live authentically, accountable to our actions and responsible for our choices, we become the hero or heroine of our own story. As such, we are to bring back the magical element of compassion to the people, which is the magical element of our own light. We are to be of service to those we love, to our community, to our mother earth and to The Divine. Our service to life then, like the hero, is the great gift of magic and renewal we bring back with us upon our return from the depths of our illness. By our struggle through our illness, we learn compassion and love and now, we serve the people through them.

Exploring further into this mythic story, we learn another significant point about our journey. When Percival rides out in his quest for the Grail, he enters the forest at a different place, a place where there is no path, a place where no one has gone before. This is a mythic invitation for us to "go into the wilderness;" to go into "the wild" and use our creativity in our healing journey. On our own quest for healing, we are expected to look where we haven't explored before. We are instructed to go into our wild places and be creative. We, as Percival, must enter the forest of our inner space from a place we have never entered before. We must ask the questions we may have never asked before about our illness, about our woundings, and about ourselves. Eventually, upon undertaking this quest, we will discover the Castle of our Holy Grail, the source of the wellspring of our creativity and self-realization deep within ourselves. It commonly exists on a road we have never taken before in a place we have never been before.

When we discover this castle, we will enter within only to find ourselves not only as Percival but also now as the wounded King bleeding from our wound of unintentional error and self-deceit. Because the King is ill, the land is ill. In mythology, a ruler is connected through his or her body to the body of the land. They are one. We are the life of the land and the life of the land is in us. We are connected to all life on earth. If the land and people are sick, we are sick. If we are sick, the land and people are sick. So to serve them, we end up serving ourselves. To heal them, we end up healing ourselves.

We can also learn a lot from the symbol of the Grail it self. It is a cup, a chalice. As the mythic tail goes, it was the cup Christ used at the last supper with his apostles. Like all cups, its message is to give life. Upon passing the Grail cup to his apostles, Jesus is to have said, "Whoso eateth my flesh, and drinketh my blood, hath eternal life."[3] A cup may store its fluid for a time, but ultimately it is required to pour it out. Its primary purpose is to serve what it holds inside so as to give nourishment, to give life. It is to share what it has been given. However, in doing this it is emptied but in its emptiness it is filled again. The grail is then the ultimate symbol of our lives in continuous creation. It demonstrates the continuous flowing of life from the Source through us into the world. We are the Grail in this mythical story as well bringing our life to the world that the world may drink. As the Grail, we learn to give fully of ourselves. In our giving, we are emptied but only to be filled again. Our quest for the Grail is not a quest to win love. It is a quest to give love. Our giving becomes an act of love and by that act we become the vessel through which life continuously flows. As it flows through us, it heals us. And so I ask again: Who will our healing serve?

A Patient Hero

A few years ago, I got a phone call from a patient I had treated successfully for a particular chronic disorder. He was a very accomplished professional athlete. He had been doing very well with his disorder which was in remission. He called to see if I had some good therapeutic ideas to give him regarding a new problem he had been experiencing. He was experiencing recurrent muscle twitching (fasciculations) occurring particularly at night in bed. He thought it might be due to an electrolyte imbalance, specifically a low magnesium level. As we talked, I began to realize his fasciculations were looking more like early symptoms of amyotrophic lateral sclerosis (ALS). I was concerned for him. I had great respect for him. He was strong and kind, courageous and humble with a good heart. I shared with him my concerns and instructed him to consult a neurologist in his local area as he lived in a different part of the country. When we next spoke, he told me my suspicions were correct and he was eventually diagnosed with ALS. A diagnosis of ALS is eventually a death certificate from progressive paralysis in four to six years.

He was recently married with his first child on the way. We talked long about the hero myth as it was exemplified in his life and through his illness. We discussed the meaning of his illness as it was manifesting in his life and his yearning for deeper self-discovery. Like the hero myth, he chose to go on his own healing quest. He left home and began his journey of self-discovery. He took a three-month van trip to the West Coast, Canada and Alaska with his wife. At the end of his journey, he found his light deep within himself and also in his new born son he called "perfect." Like the hero he is, he has returned from his journey to give back to his people the gift he had found in himself, his gift of compassion. He has begun a nonprofit organization to raise awareness about ALS and to provide help to individuals with neuromuscular diseases or injuries by using leading-edge technology, equipment and services. He has recently been quoted to say, "I think I've always lived with some purpose and had some intentions. That's not going to change because of my illness. The opportunity to inspire other people to live with purpose is a great one." In all respects, he is healed and he is healing his people. He is living the myth. He is a living hero.

My Patient Hero

My mother was always a strong woman, a foundational rock in our family. In 2006 she had a stroke while visiting my cousin in Florida with my father who was already seriously confused from his progressing dementia. She was 84 at the time. I don't know how she did it, but she carted my father off on a plane and they flew off together to see my cousin. One morning back in Seattle, I was awakened by a call from my cousin. Mom had a stroke and I needed to call the Emergency Room ASAP. I called and spoke with the doctor. I had a decision to make that could either save my mother's life or kill her. I made the decision to go ahead with the anticoagulant medication and immediately jumped on a plane. In the week that followed, my mother came through like a trooper with only mild paralysis and a mild speech impediment. She had grandchildren and my father to care for. She was still on her mission of serving and she wouldn't let something like this interfere with that mission. After a few more weeks, I flew out to Florida again to get my parents and escort them back home.

For two more years my mother continued caring for all of us including my ailing father who now, was getting to be too much for her to handle. They were a unit; married 63 years. They did everything together. One day while my wife and I were painting our living room, I brought mom over to direct the job. Literally overnight her legs were swollen and her abdomen was distended. She was having trouble breathing. I knew what was going on. We took her into the hospital that day and she was admitted for evaluation. She was diagnosed with ovarian cancer and began chemotherapy. Through her treatment she began to realize the struggle I was having with managing her care and my father's care. She knew my father had to be moved to a special care unit without her. I went to the hospital one day between patients at the office. I was stressed that day attempting to manage her care, my father's care, my parents' financial matters, my practice and, my family. Somehow, that day, she looked at me like she had never looked at me before. She saw my struggle and something changed in her. She realized there was little left for her to do and she couldn't be of service anymore. The following day I was called by her doctor and told she was going into kidney and heart failure. Her heart was broken. She never wanted to be a burden to anyone.

I rushed to the hospital to find my mother alone in a room attached to a morphine IV pump. She was slowly progressing into complete failure but was fully conscious and conversational. My family and I gathered around her bed and for ten out of thirteen hours she was fully with us. We held her, said goodbye to her, remembered so many special times with her. She was in pain and she knew she was dying yet she joked and laughed and gave us instruction about taking care of each other. She was strong to the last second of her life. She knew even in her death she would be caring for us. She was and is a hero to us all. She taught us how to face death with courage. This is what heroes do. On the evening of July eighth, 2008, my life-long patient hero died; my mother died.

Dr. Patrick Donovan

Victim or Hero?

In our healing journey through illness, we have the power to choose how we will experience it and what story will be told of us. Will our story be one of heroism and courage; one of authenticity and truth? Or will our story be one of passivity, stagnation and ennui; one of victimization and illusion? My patient with ALS and my mother chose stories of heroism when faced with their illness and death as have so many of my patients. I have been made stronger by their stories. I have been given courage and guidance by the way they have lived their stories. Their stories have given me instructions on how to follow the thread of my own hero path. Their lives have become a roadmap for me and all who know them; a roadmap to study when we are faced with our own healing journey. When our time comes and we choose to follow their map and their instruction, "where we had thought to find an abomination, we shall find a god; where we had thought to slay another, we shall slay ourselves; where we had thought to travel outward, we shall come to the center of our own existence; where we had thought to be alone, we shall be with all the world." Where we had thought to be ill, we will be healed.

References

1. Neumann E: *The Origins and History of Consciousness.* Princeton University Press, 1954; 149
2. Campbell J: *The Hero With A Thousand Faces.* Princeton University Press, 1973; 25
3. John 6:54. *King James Bible* (Cambridge Ed.)

Chapter Ten

The Sovereignty of Self

"The sovereignty of one's self over one's self is called Liberty."
(*Albert Pike*)

"You can be a thousand different women. It's your choice
which one you want to be. It's about freedom and sovereignty.
You celebrate who you are. You say, 'This is my kingdom.'"
(*Salma Hayek*)

"If the choice were made, one for us to lose our sovereignty
and become a member of the Commonwealth or remain
with our sovereignty and lose the membership of the
Commonwealth, I would say let the Commonwealth go."
(*Robert Mugabe*)

The Oxygen Mask

It is late and you just made it to the gate on time with your
two young children. You board the plane with the first
calling because you have children and it takes time to get
them situated and seated. You sit on the aisle seat with your two
children sitting in the window and center seats. Finally the plane
is fully boarded and it begins to taxi. You are nervous, worried
for the safety of your children. They are all you have and you love
them dearly. Then, the flight attendant introduces the flight staff
and begins the instructions. "In case of an emergency, the oxygen
masks are employed from the overhead compartment above you,"

she states. Then she goes on to instruct you to put YOUR mask on first and secure it tightly before you help your children put on their masks. "What!" You think to yourself. "How could that be? Surely she is mistaking. I must take care of my children first. They come before me." Then she further explains the rationale for this safety instruction. "If the compartment loses oxygen rapidly," she explains, "parents may black out before being able to help their children secure their masks and then no one is safe."

One of the hardest of concepts for many of us to understand is the concept of self-importance. In our social structure, we are led to believe it means selfishness. It does not. If we are unhealthy and incapable of serving those we love we will then be failing them. The degree to which we fail them is then proportionate to the degree to which we are incapacitated and failing ourselves. There is something logical about taking care of ourselves first if we are going to be of service to others. This is not being selfish. It is the logic of self-care and comes from loving ourselves enough to take care of ourselves so that we may be fully present for those whom we love.

In my many years of observing and studying the nature of illness, I have come to realize so much of its causative dysfunction, occurring both personally and societally, arises from our inability to love ourselves unconditionally. If we recall for instance, my earlier description of the energetic or consciousness theme underlying autoimmune disorders, it is one of self-criticism and self-directed anger . . . "self attacking self." This does not arise from an internal energetic of loving one's self. It arises from an internal energetic of contempt for one's self on some deep level. As we study the medical literature and disease trends over the past one hundred years or so of "modernization" of our society, we quickly see there has been a marked increase in autoimmune illnesses throughout the "Western Civilized World." It is no wonder we see this trend as it is perpetuated by a socio-religious culture of contempt and disdain for the sovereignty and freedom of the human soul, especially if that soul is female. Hence, the more autoimmune disorders commonly occurring in women than in men.

Mea Culpa, Mea Culpa, Mea Maxima Culpa

Our Western Civilized World has been primed, ripened and fertilized with more than two thousand years of the doctrine of *original sin*, the *fall of man*, the *corruption of nature*, the *inequality of women*, and the *unworthiness and guilt* of the sinful self. For, as Romans 3:23 tells us "All have sinned and fall short of the glory of God." This doctrine is born from the local, hunter-dominator tribal, traditions of the Middle East. It is a doctrine that promotes a single-parented familial patriarchal hierarchy as its metaphorical structure for spiritual practice and societal law. At the top of this hierarchy rules a stern, anthropomorphic, patriarchal Godhead (*Yahweh or Allah*) who rules over His less than worthy, commonly disobedient children (us) who's original parents (Adam and Eve) already sinned terribly against the Lord (*original sin*) eternally staining all of our souls with their sin even before we are born. They were banished from the Garden of Eden for eating an apple from the Tree of Knowledge of Good and Evil. In a sense, they were banished for choosing knowledge over ignorance; freedom over slavery by being able to discern and discriminate between "good and evil" so that they might be free to choose for themselves.

Further, this patriarchal Godhead rules from His throne far up in heaven separate from His creation and endlessly struggles against all the other gods of the world for domination. This familial hierarchy is a useful metaphorical model to project into our collective consciousness when control is of primary importance. Control of any one of us is easy when we identify with the unworthy, disobedient, and sinful children of this metaphorical model fearing our Father's retribution (God-fearing) at any moment we make the "wrong" decision. It is then in our best interest to not risk making that decision and please our father and keep him happy lest we be punished or lose his favor and blessing. As a child, our primary concern is worthiness of our father's blessing. Our worthiness is based on obedience to the rules of the house and not on the beauty and creative novelty of our own being. Whoever is in charge of God's dispensation of justice (the church, the government, etc.) is in control. To question our Father or the rationality and practicality of His rules/laws in any way is to risk his wrath and so, we obey without question and call it faith. This is not freedom and it certainly stands in blatant opposition to free choice and the espoused doctrine of "free will."

Does this system of belief make you feel vitally connected to an omnipresent loving Divine Source through an intimate, personal, and nurturing relationship that encourages self-expression, self-discovery, and creativity? Does this feel like a permissive relationship through which you are encouraged to live your life fully and be responsible for the unfolding of your own path of destiny? It certainly doesn't for me! It makes me feel worthless and guilty for being who I am, worried that every choice I make may be the "wrong choice" incurring God's wrath. So, with this guilt and worry, I would be forced to live a restrictive cautious life fearful of taking any risks at all that may cause me to "step out of the box" or "outside of my comfort zone" to be explorationally creative and discover my own truth. In this state of living, I would live a less than creative existence; an existence devoid of my own freedom of expression and self-discovery.

It is no wonder why I see so much neurosis and anxiety disorders underlying the illnesses of my patients who are raised in our modern Western World under such a restrictive doctrine of belief. As a matter of fact, I have seen this belief system of obedient unworthiness and fear of condemnation, contribute much to the dysfunctional energetics of illness and denial in most of my patients. But, to my disbelief, they often desperately hold on to it because it keeps them safe from being truly free and accountable . . . from being truly sovereign and creative. Instead, they would rather proclaim, "Mea culpa, mea culpa, mea maxima culpa! (It is my fault! It is my fault. It is my most grievous fault!). Father please forgive me for I have sinned and am so unworthy of your love!" There is no loving self unconditionally here. With this proclamation, they can now be off the hook of having to be fully free and accountable; to be fully dynamic, authentic, and self-creative.

Permission to Be

I was a mouthy, know-it-all teenager in high-school always questioning authority. I never felt motivated to do more than I needed to do to pass my classes. But when I started my first day of tenth grade English, I became motivated. It wasn't about me just deciding to change on my own. It was all about something my tenth grade English teacher told me and my fellow students on that first day of class. She said, "All of you start this class with an A. It is your choice what you do with that A. You can keep it or lose it. However, I see all of you in this class as talented students with something of great value to teach us and to offer to the world; something specific and special to each one of you. I want to give all of you the freedom and encouragement in this class to discover what that is and how you can best share it." Wow! I was all of the sudden important and of value and not just this flunky teenager who knew nothing. I wrote like I never wrote before in this class . . . poetry, pros, etc. I had something of value to share, something to say about the world and how I saw it. Someone finally gave me permission to discover "me" and be who I was while giving me the freedom to express it. Someone told me I had value and I mattered in this world, not what I shouldn't do, shouldn't say, or shouldn't be. Now, here I am, healing myself and doing my best to contribute to the healing of the world with my writing because I was allowed to discover my sixteen-year old self and bring it creatively out into the world. This healed me on some deep level because this permissive canon of recognizing the unlimited potential in ourselves and each other, while also providing the platform to realize it, is transformative. It heals us. It cultivates hope and encourages the creative expression and unfoldment of ourselves. It allows us to become the hero or heroine of our own story.

Our creativity and freedom of expression is crucial to our health and our healing journey as I have discussed earlier. We are not well as a person or a society when we cannot, within the bounds of mutual respect for each other's sovereignty, freely create and self-express while allowing others their creative self-expression as well. Further, such a level of creativity and self-expression requires of us to know ourselves. It also requires of us to conquer our fear of fully living our path of destiny and the freedom and responsibility it brings us. Are you ready for this? Are you strong and centered enough in your own self to accept the many different possibilities, expressions, and conflicting ideas that may arise in such a freely expressive environment while at the same time allowing all others their due sovereignty and freedom of expression?

Over my many years of patient interactions, I have come to measure the health of a person as well as the health of a community or society, by the degree to which they can be freely creative and expressive of themselves, dialoging and sharing ideas between each other while not being intimidated or threatened by other differing thoughts, concepts, and criticisms. As a matter of fact, the free expression and open dialogue of such differing thoughts and ideas has historically been the very brewing pot that has fermented and catalyzed the growth and human evolution of our consciousness and awareness as individuals and as a society. This free and open dialogue is the foundation stone of democracy and the charge of our universities. However, it is not possible in a society where individual sovereignty and freedom of expression is discouraged, denied, or repudiated. It is not encouraged when the leading system of belief and social structure is one of unworthiness and guilt steeped in a hierarchical structure of ruler ship over the many by the chosen few. Isn't it to go something like this: Of the people; By the people; For the people?

The Sovereign Hero

As we discovered in the previous chapter, the way to our healing is found by following the thread of the hero path. But as we follow that thread, as it takes us through our healing journey, we quickly realize *sovereignty of self* is the most relevant aspect of this hero path and therefore of our healing. This path demands of each one of us that we claim and live fully our inherent sovereignty as a human soul. What is sovereignty and what does it mean to live it fully? Well, as I like to simply define it, sovereignty, in a generalized sense, is the quality of being fully free; free to be who we were born to be. In a more specific sense, for us to be sovereign is for us to exercise our right of domain and power over ourselves and our own lives and no one else's lives, while exercising our freedom of choice. Sovereignty assures us our individuality. Most importantly, however, *sovereignty honors life's prime directive of "free choice"* and as a result of that free choice, it also *honors the emergence of creativity and "optimal diversity."*

Life loves diversity! Every biologist knows this. The more diverse a living system is, the healthier it is and the healthier it is, the more creative and dynamic it is. As a matter of fact, diversity is a special form of creativity, as I discussed in my book, *The Face of Consciousness*. It assures the maximal unfolding of all the possibilities of identity and relationship and every opportunity to grow into greater richness and variety. Therefore, on a more personal level, sovereignty allows us the freedom and opportunity to be optimally creative while assuring us the maximal unfolding of all of our individual possibilities of identity and relationship and every opportunity for us to grow into a richer and more dynamic individual. *Sovereignty offers us our healing and gives us our medicine.*

At this point we might ask ourselves, "What are the requirements of us to live as sovereign beings?" To live as a sovereign being, I believe, requires of us to live fully the truth of "who" we are while being fully responsible for and accountable to our own actions, words, thoughts, and choices. To be sovereign, is to live authentically and be "the captain of our own ship." I think it also requires of us the respect of all other's sovereignty and freedom of expression as well. We do this by not imposing "our" domain and control upon anyone else. The exception to this is with our children. We certainly must impose our domain upon them at first as they are initially an extension of ourselves and unable to realize their own sovereignty early on. Then slowly, as they grow, mature, and develop into a responsible adult, we slowly release them from our dominion allowing them their own sovereignty. You may also be wondering, "How do we acquire our sovereignty?" Here, again, the instruction to discovering our sovereignty is found in the same instruction given to us for discovering our healing as I have attempted to elucidate in this book. It is found in the following of the thread of the Hero path.

If we follow the thread of the hero path we quickly find it leads us into our sovereignty by compelling us to: 1) leave the comfort, safety, and security of the familiar, common norms and constructs of home, family, society, and beliefs; 2) break new ground (step outside of the box) for ourselves and the overall human journey of evolving consciousness; 3) enter the wilderness at a different place, a place where there is no path, a place where no one has gone before; 4) die to our old ways of living and thinking that no longer serve our continued growth and evolution, and; 5) resurrect from the death of our limited self into the fullness of our greater self, our sovereign self. This sovereign self that resurrects is our healed self, our greater self that knows who we are and why we are here. When, like the hero, we arise into our sovereignty, no one and nothing outside of us can then defeat us or take from us the truth of who we are. But be warned, the truly sovereign individuals throughout history, the many heroes and heroines of our world, have been commonly crucified, murdered, and sacrificed on the societal thrones and alters of fear and control; murdered by the very people they have come to serve and come to set free. A sovereign individual is a free individual and this is a threat to those of us who would control and to those of us who live in fear and denial.

A free and sovereign individual, just by virtue of his/her being alive, constantly reminds us of our failures and the work we need yet to do to overcome our own deep fears of living. This is an embarrassment to our egoic self and so we strive to eliminate that embarrassment instead of striving to free ourselves. We then conspire and contrive to find some reason or excuse to kill our heroes and so we do. Also, a free and sovereign individual cannot be easily controlled. So, for those of us who strive to control others in the face of our own weaknesses and fear, a sovereign individual is a threat to our construct of control and must be removed. In each case, after we eliminate the threat and embarrassment of such an individual, we then put that person on a pedestal and honor him/her for their sovereignty and heroism because now we are safe and we can envy them their sovereignty in the privacy of our own little and shrinking spaces of authenticity. In truth we fear our freedom because it demands of us our full and authentic participation in life as a fully creative, self-realized and self-actualized human being. In truth we fear our healing because it demands of us the same. Our healing demands of us to be all we were born to be to our fullest and to be it in a way in which we serve life. I call upon each one of us as I call upon myself to proclaim our individual sovereignty and BE the medicine we bring to the world.

CPSIA information can be obtained at www.ICGtesting.com
Printed in the USA
LVOW12s1214201113

362074LV00001B/87/P